Teaching Orthopaedics

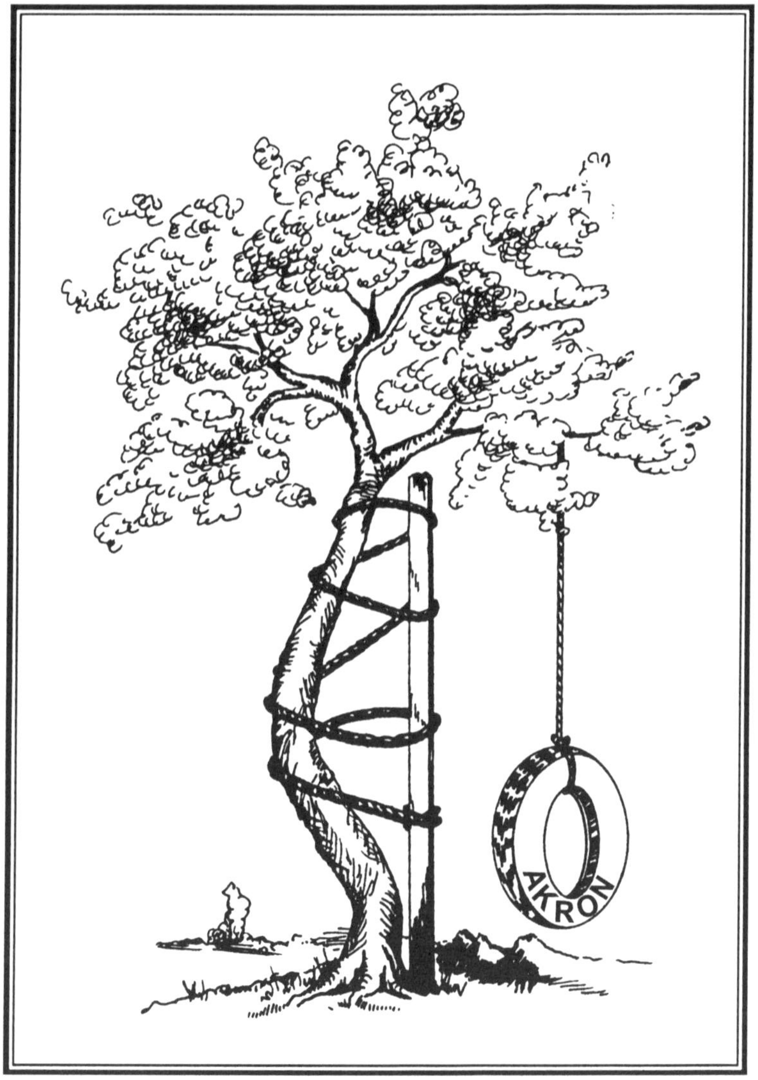

in the Rubber City

Priscilla M. Harding

Layout and Design by:
Stephen H. Paschen

ISBN 0-9671505-0-7

Cover Graphic: Nicholas Andre's Tree of Orthopaedics

In 1741, Nicholas Andre published *L'Orthopedie*, the first book devoted exclusively to orthopaedic surgery. He wrote his book "to teach the different methods of preventing and correcting the deformities of children." For more than 250 years, his Tree of Orthopaedics, bent and bowed, but held fast to a strong stake to straighten its trunk, has symbolized the orthopaedic surgeon's prime task -- restoring normal function. The "Akron" automobile tire, suspended from Andre's Tree of Orthopaedics, identifies and personalizes our story, which is *Teaching Orthopaedics in the Rubber City*.

Harding, Priscilla M. Harding
Teaching Orthopaedics in the Rubber City

Photographs provided by Summa Health System, The University of Akron Archives, Children's Hospital Medical Center, Akron General Medical Center.

Bibliography

Includes Index

1. 1892-1945, Early Teachers 2. 1946-1969, Setting the Foundation
3. 1970-1982, Building An Academic Base
4. 1983-1997, A New, Exciting Golden Era 5. Having Their Say.
Appendix.

Printed and Bound by Sheridan Books, Chelsea, Michigan

Teaching Orthopaedics in the Rubber City

By Priscilla M. Harding

Table of Contents

i Foreword

iii Acknowledgments

v Introduction

1 Chapter One
1892-1945, Early Teachers

25 Chapter Two
1946-1969, Setting the Foundation

49 Chapter Three
1970-1982, Building An Academic Base

75 Chapter Four
1983-1997, A New, Exciting Golden Era

93 Chapter Five
Having Their Say

119 Appendix

131 Bibliography

135 Index

Foreword

Orthopaedic resident education in Akron has grown through the efforts of numerous innovative and productive surgeons, whose clinical excellence has been passed down to the present generation.

To date, the history of the department has not been formally recorded. However, we are fortunate that many physicians who have trained the present group of clinicians are still willing and able to recreate the chronology and the significant events from our past that have helped to shape the present department.

There is no history that will do justice to all who have given their life's work to the care of others and to training of young residents. To those who have been unintentionally slighted I offer my sincere apology because our heritage would not be as strong as it is without the contribution of all who unselfishly have contributed many hours to the growth and development of this department.

It is my hope that all future residents will benefit from our heritage and realize that "Yesterday's Professors" were some of the most creative and insightful individuals that have had the privilege to serve as guardians of life and limb.

Hopefully, the changes in the health care system that lie ahead will not diminish our role as clinicians, educators and researchers. With proper vision and dedication, present department members will continue the pursuit of excellence in order that future generations will look favorably upon our efforts and remember us with the fondness and reverence with which we hold our mentors whose deeds will be described in this volume.

J. Patrick Flanagan, M.D.
Chairman, Department of Orthopaedics
Summa Health System

Acknowledgments

I owe many thanks to Akron's orthopaedic surgeons, nurses, and support staff, some of whom had been gathering material for a souvenir manuscript for a year before I came on the scene. J. Patrick Flanagan, Chairman of the Department of Orthopaedic Surgery at Summa Health System, wrote to classmates and colleagues across the country in 1994, reminding them of the upcoming fiftieth anniversary of City/Children's orthopaedic residency program and requesting their reminiscences. William M. Davis, retired orthopaedic surgeon, spearheaded these efforts and became a familiar presence in Summa's Office of Orthopaedic Administration at St. Thomas Hospital. Jeff Gardner, the research assistant in those early days, dug into newspaper files and hospital records and unearthed valuable nuggets of information. Carol Larsen, Administrative Assistant to Ed Pfeiffer, then the Administrative Director of Orthopaedic Services at Summa, oversaw this growing mass of material and could produce a requested paper in the twinkling of an eye.

Information was sometimes difficult to obtain, however; Jeff accepted a new job in 1995, and time overwhelmed the team. The orthopaedic residency's golden anniversary celebration was only fifteen months away when, in June 1995, I joined this group. Support personnel are at the heart of any enterprise. They arranged interviews and gathered material for me at each of the hospitals and I appreciate it. Bill Davis was very helpful throughout that hectic fifteen months, always available, very informative. I interviewed a number of orthopaedists, some of whom also contributed papers. Their contributions are listed in the bibliography and I thank them for educating me about their specialty. Jean Morton, R.N., wrote a paper presenting the orthopaedic nurse's viewpoint and I spent a delightful couple of hours chatting with Mrs. Morton about her career at City Hospital. Walter A. Hoyt, Jr., retired Chairman of City Hospital's Department of Orthopaedic Surgery, gave me insight into the impact national developments have had on these community hospital programs.

When it was decided to turn the manuscript into a book, I literally "moved across the hall" at St. Thomas Hospital and set up shop in the Department of Orthopaedic Surgery where Summa's orthopaedic residency program is located. In this final phase of the project, I've had the good fortune to work with Penny La Bate, Senior Administrative Secretary, and Delphia

Rutherford, Administrative Secretary. Both have a large store of knowledge about orthopaedics and I deeply appreciate all their help. I owe a big debt of gratitude to Dr. Hoyt. He gave me the benefit of his long experience in orthopaedic education and, as the book developed, went through two manuscript revisions with grace, good humor, and an expert eye. Finally, my friend, Barbara E. Clements, Professor of History at the University of Akron, critiqued the fourth revision of the manuscript. Her astute questions and pointed comments cut through the foggy patches, saved me from several literary pratfalls, and truly helped me make *Teaching Orthopaedics in the Rubber City* a much better book than it would have been otherwise.

Introduction

"Dintism"

"Teaching Orthopaedics in the Rubber City" began "in house" in 1993, or thereabouts, with the aim of producing a souvenir manuscript relating how three generations of physicians worked together to build Akron's orthopaedic residency programs. The impetus for this project was the rapidly approaching fiftieth anniversary (in October 1996) of City/Children's Hospitals' residency in orthopaedic surgery. In June 1995, I joined a team of doctors and support staff, gathered material, interviewed orthopaedists, and completed a manuscript in time for the golden anniversary celebration. Shortly after the party, it was decided to turn the souvenir manuscript into a book.

Why write a local history about such an esoteric subject as teaching the specialty of orthopaedic surgery? For one thing, the Akron experience exemplifies the exponential growth of scientific medicine and graduate education in the twentieth century - with a twist. Akron had no medical school until the seventies. It never has had a "university hospital" of the sort usually associated with medical education. Given this lack of academic accouterments, the city seems an unlikely place to find top-notch residencies in orthopaedic surgery. And yet, here they are, developed by physicians who grew with their specialty. They continued their education, attended conferences, did research, brought back procedures and instruments, and, in three generations, progressed from skilled trauma surgeons to board-certified specialists in orthopaedic surgery.

Postgraduate (residency) education in medicine came about because medical knowledge expanded so enormously in the twentieth century. Approximately twenty-five medical schools in the United States offered residencies in orthopaedics in the 1930's. Interest in the specialty grew dramatically following World War II, and the number of residencies in orthopaedic surgery mushroomed to 238, some in community hospitals such as those in Akron that had no connection to a medical school. Practitioners established two programs in Akron, Ohio, at City Hospital (now Summa Health System) in 1946, and, at Akron General Hospital (now Akron General Medical Center) in 1957.

Strong individuals built these residencies, men who perceived a challenge as an opportunity. In 1964, for instance, they took up the challenge of teaching orthopaedic basic science (biomechanics) in Akron instead of sending their residents to the University of Pennsylvania's Graduate School of

Medicine for nine months. In so doing, these clinicians gained valuable experience in medicine's academic side. The character of the founders provides an even more important element in the success of these programs, however. Two surgeons of the first generation of teachers, Walter A. Hoyt, Sr. and Fowler B. Roberts, were instrumental in founding Akron's first orthopaedic surgery residency at City and Children's. Dr. Roberts joined second generation teachers, Donald I. Minnig, Edwin L. Mollin, and Harry O'Dell, all senior attendings at Akron General Hospital, in establishing that orthopaedic residency.

These men, and others, created a collegial atmosphere that continues today. As one of the current generation, Tom Bear, says, "We all excel, we all try to be the best, we all are after our share of the market. But, we're all colleagues in this town." This collegial attitude has benefitted patients for nearly a century and will continue for years to come. The physicians in *Teaching Orthopaedics in the Rubber City* explore the orthopaedic landscape, absorb the latest developments in their profession, and share this knowledge with their colleagues.

Orthopaedic surgery's fund of knowledge comes to Akron from all over the world and it has expanded so rapidly over the last half century that the task of simply "keeping up" is never ending. Sometimes, the true realization of knowledge gained dawns much later, such as with Bill Davis, who originally disliked assisting a super-meticulous hand surgeon named Sterling Bunnell. Other times, as Zouhair Yassine discovered, what seems a perfect site for a skiing vacation can also yield important new methods of setting fractures. And, knowledge has its dangers. Whit Ewing read *The Atlas of Arthroscopy* by Dr. Masake Watanabe, decided it was the "logical way to establish a correct diagnosis of knee joint pathology," and risked his eyesight to learn the technique. Time and again, these physicians have stumbled onto knowledge, made it their own, and passed it along. They know they can never stop learning because knowledge is what keeps them ahead of the game in the world of medicine.

World renowned cellist Lynn Harrell discovered early in his career what it takes to stay ahead of the game in the world of music and, a few years ago, he shared the secret with graduates of the Cleveland Institute of Music. A member of the Cleveland Symphony Orchestra at age eighteen, Harrell considered himself "a finished product. Now I had arrived. All the hard work was behind me." Maestro George Szell asked him to stay behind during a rehearsal break, seized the young cellist's bow arm, and whipped the bow across the strings with such force, the cello shrieked. "You don't contribute," Szell roared. "You don't know anything. You're not prepared. You just float along down the stream. You never know how the music goes."

Then the taskmaster became the teacher. Szell, Harrell said, "taught me respect for the creative force behind a great piece of music. He taught me respect for my fellow musicians...told me about studying the score, about practicing music and not just technique; about learning to hear the rest of the music, to study the architecture of a piece, the lines weaving through it in the individual instruments...."

"The key is simple," Harrell told the graduates, "you just have to keep going. It isn't a competition. It's only about yourself, about one practice day after another, about forcing yourself to understand that you will never understand it all. The British have a term which I have just discovered. It's called dintism. 'How did he get that job?' I asked about a colleague. "Oh, dintism," came the answer. It is - it was explained to me - 'by sheer dint of doing it.' Of doing it with good will and effort day after day, year after year. Of not giving up."

Dintism operates in any profession, or, for that matter, in life. The bar of knowledge continually rises, the studying goes on, research continues, and the teacher often becomes the student. Those who teach orthopaedics in the Rubber City understand this very well. This is their story.

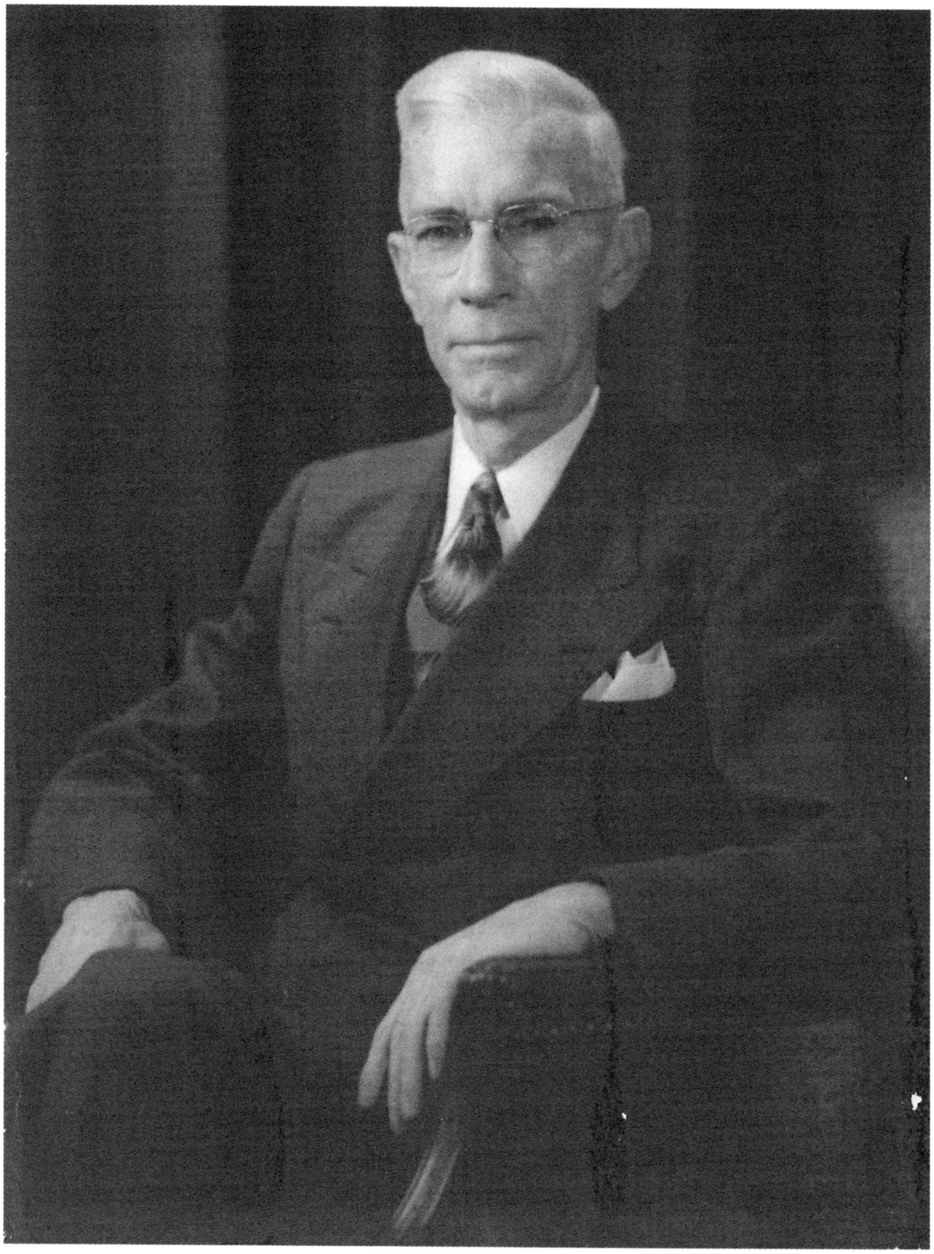

Walter A. Hoyt, Sr.: Dr. Hoyt came to Akron in 1916 to organize and chair Northeastern Ohio's first Department of Orthopaedic Surgery at Akron's Children's Hospital. In 1920, he was appointed to the Advisory Board of Ohio's newly formed Society for Crippled Children, which is concerned with the physical and psychological management of pediatric orthopaedic problems. In 1937, he was appointed to the Orthopaedic Council of the National Foundation for Infantile Paralysis, the first nationwide organization dedicated to eliminating a specific disease. As Chief of Akron City Hospital's Division of Orthopaedic Surgery, he was instrumental in developing City's Orthopaedic Residency program, which was approved in 1947. A fine clinician, researcher, and teacher, Dr. Hoyt's career is a model of scientific medical practice in the first half of the twentieth century.

Photograph supplied by W. A. Hoyt, Jr.

Chapter One

1892-1945, Early Teachers

Orthopaedics, like all fields of modern medicine, is a product of the last hundred years of extraordinary progress in scientific understanding and technological innovation. American orthopaedics was recognized as a distinct surgical specialty by 1920 and from that time through 1945, thirteen surgeons did orthopaedic work in Akron, Ohio: Millard C. Beyer, I.R. Birnbaum, George Bischoff, Harold R. Conn, Adrian E. Davis, Patrick C. Doran, Walter A. Hoyt, Sr., Rey V. Luce, Donald I. Minnig, Edwin L. Mollin, William A. Parks, Fowler B. Roberts, and Carl Steinke. Over the years, these men gained a wealth of experience treating the crippled child, the injured factory worker, the wounded soldier, experience they shared with the hospitals' general surgery residents. When the time came in 1946 to organize a combined orthopaedic residency program at Children's and City Hospitals, the Rubber City possessed a cadre of experienced surgeon/teachers, eager to pass along their knowledge of orthopaedics to a new generation.

One of these early teachers, Walter Asahel Hoyt, Sr., M.D., came to Akron in 1916 at the invitation of William S. Chase, M.D., Chief of Staff at Children's Hospital. Orthopaedic surgeons were making significant progress treating the crippled child in those days. Chase's hospital had a Ward for Crippled Children and now the Chief of Staff sought an experienced, knowledgeable surgeon to establish a full-fledged Department of Orthopaedic Surgery at Children's. A 1911 graduate of The University of Michigan Medical School, Hoyt was qualified, having completed five years of postgraduate medical education (the length of today's orthopaedic residency) as an assistant to Michigan's Professor of Surgery, Charles B. Nancrede. "They didn't want to lose him [at the University of Michigan]," Hoyt's son recalled years later, "but, Dr. Chase made him an offer he couldn't refuse." Chase's enticing challenge, building a department of orthopaedics, combined with the necessity of providing for a growing family, persuaded the young surgeon to strike out on his own.

Hoyt's teacher, Charles B. Nancrede, an 1869 graduate of the University of Pennsylvania's School of Medicine, exemplifies the turn-of-the-century scientific medical practitioner. As a junior attending physician at Philadelphia's Episcopal Hospital, he was one of the first surgeons in the city to adopt antiseptic and aseptic surgery. Nancrede did research on a wide range of subjects publishing several articles annually in various local [Philadelphia] journals.

(Orthopaedic topics include "pathology of the shoulder joint," "fractures of the neck of the humerus," "tumor of the scapula," and "fracture of the ankle joint.")

In 1889, Victor Vaughan, M.D., Dean of the University of Michigan's Medical School, recruited Nancrede to come to Ann Arbor and build a Department of Surgery, which he did, retiring in 1917. During Nancrede's tour at Michigan, American medical education changed appreciably. It was no longer a few months of lectures followed by apprenticeship to a private practitioner; now, hospital experience and basic science were medical curriculum mainstays. W.A. Hoyt, Sr. was a second year medical student at Michigan in 1909 when Abraham Flexner, a layman representing the Carnegie Foundation for the Advancement of Teaching, accompanied by the secretary of the American Medical Association's Council on Medical Education, inspected the school, which had the first university hospital in the nation. In his report, *Medical Education in the United States and Canada*, Flexner wrote that

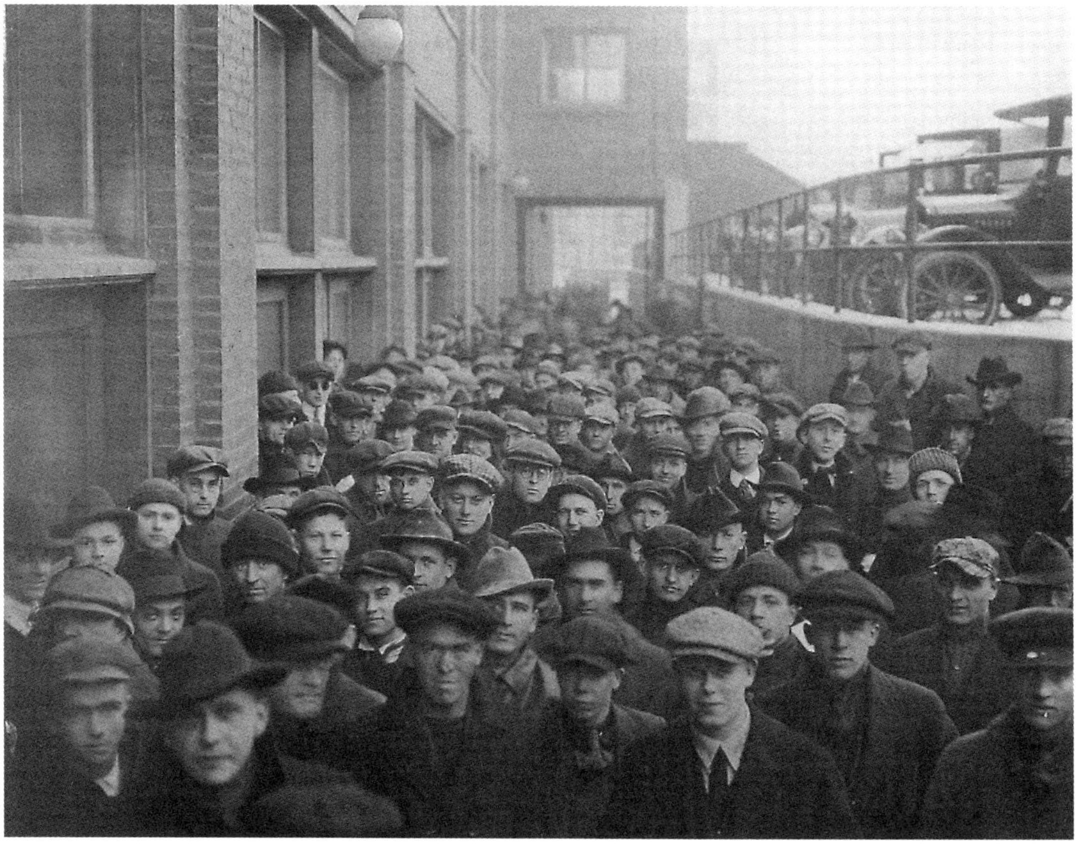

Shift change at Goodyear in the late teens. So scarce was Akron housing in those days that rubber workers rented sleeping rooms in shifts. **University of Akron Archives**

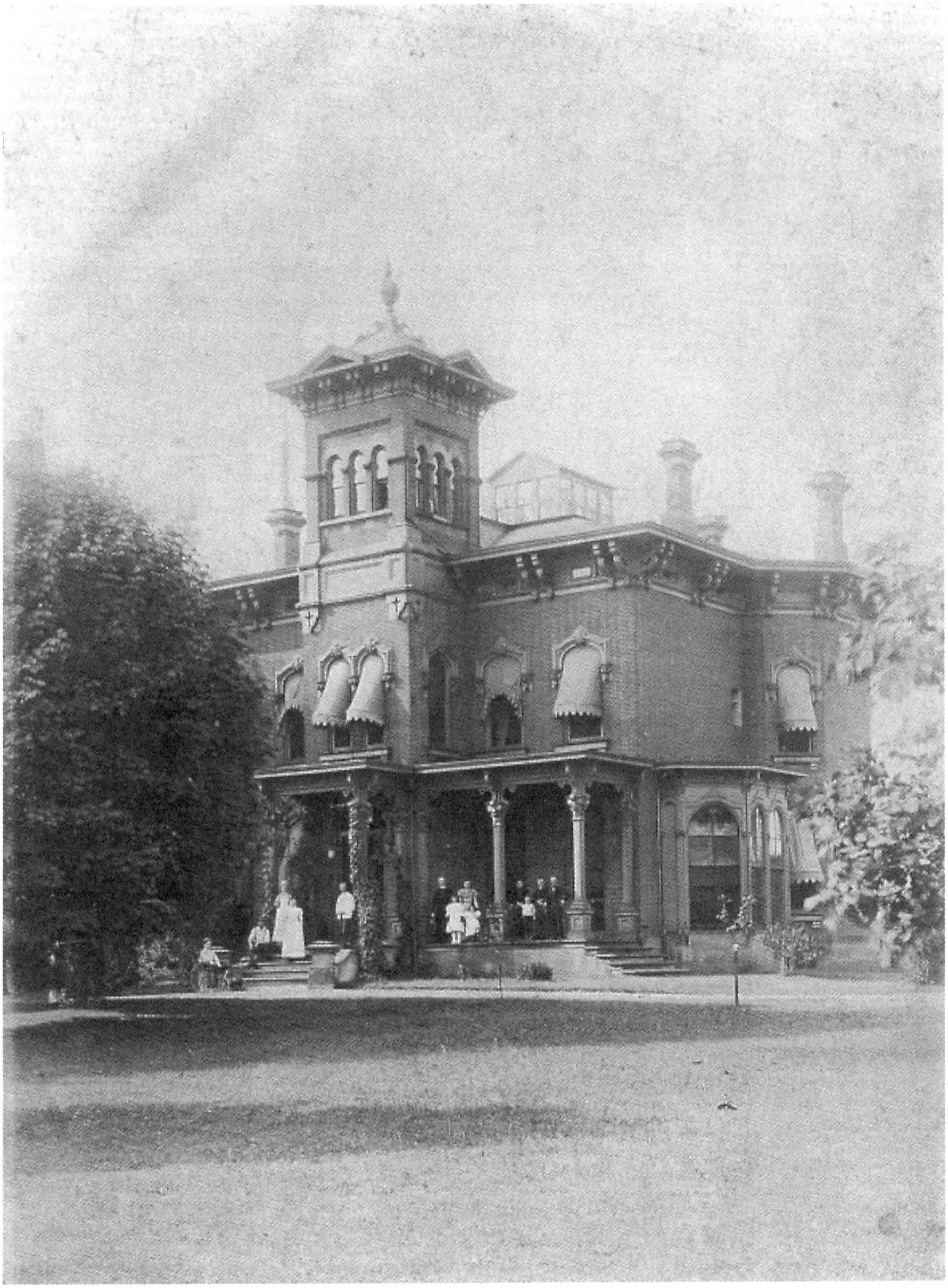

Staff and patients pose for a photo in c.1895 on the steps and porch of the Bartges house, Akron City Hospital's first home.
University of Akron Archives

"[Michigan] is fortunate in the possession of its own hospital, every case in which can be used for the purposes of instruction." According to Horace W. Davenport, Ph.D., author of *Fifty Years of Medicine at the University of*

Michigan, 1891-1941, Nancrede's "most successful teaching was at the operating table or at the bedside...[In the operating room] he worked [as] quickly as the condition of the patient would permit. He kept the patient warm, and he tried to avoid shock by keeping the patient's head low...He was particularly solicitous in his after-care, and he frequently stayed in the hospital all night to observe a patient. He changed the dressings himself." Now, thanks to Dr. Chase, one of Nancrede's senior assistants would bring these lessons, and more, to Akron.

The Hoyt family's new home was very different from the quiet university town of Ann Arbor. Akron was the Rubber Capital of the World in 1916, a smoky, gritty mill town, suffused with an acrid odor dubbed "the smell of money." Memorial Day geraniums planted at East Akron Cemetery, across Market Street from one of the thriving rubber factories, turned ash-grey in hours then, their blooms peppered with grit.

Rubber company founders, Harvey Firestone, Sr., and Frank and Charles Seiberling of Goodyear, contributed generously to Akron's hospitals. George Todd Perkins, one of those who brought Dr. Benjamin Goodrich to town, thereby launching Akron's rubber industry, was Children's Hospital's most generous benefactor in its early days. Akron's three adult hospitals followed the city's population. City Hospital is in the east part of town, Peoples (Akron General Medical Center) in the west, and St. Thomas Hospital lies across the Little Cuyahoga River Valley, just north of downtown.

City Hospital opened in 1892 on East Market Street, then a fashionable avenue lined with elegant homes. Dr. Samuel Bartges's stately home, which housed City, was "one of the most substantial and prominent structures in Akron," according to the *Akron Beacon and Republican.* City soon outgrew the mansion and its annex (added in 1898), and in 1904, increased its capacity from twenty-one to seventy beds when it opened a brand new hospital east of the Bartges mansion. That structure contains administrative offices today, its upper stories barely visible among the many additions on the current hospi-

> Injuries from traffic accidents, today so commonplace they rarely make the papers, are a source of much orthopaedic work. Automobile driving was a new experience when, on a bright May Sunday in 1918, fledgling drivers and incautious pedestrians combined to "make street travel a constant race with death," according to the *Akron Beacon Journal.* Six traffic accidents left one man dead, a three-year-old in Children's Hospital, two adults in City, two more treated at Peoples and released, and one not requiring treatment. In a burst of hyperbole, the *Beacon* reporter said that "speeding automobiles, careless drivers, equally careless pedestrians, reckless trolley motormen, incompetents operating gasoline driven vehicles, and a police force [inadequate] to curb the existing conditions are fast making the death risk on Akron's streets more dangerous than life in the front line trenches (in World War I)."

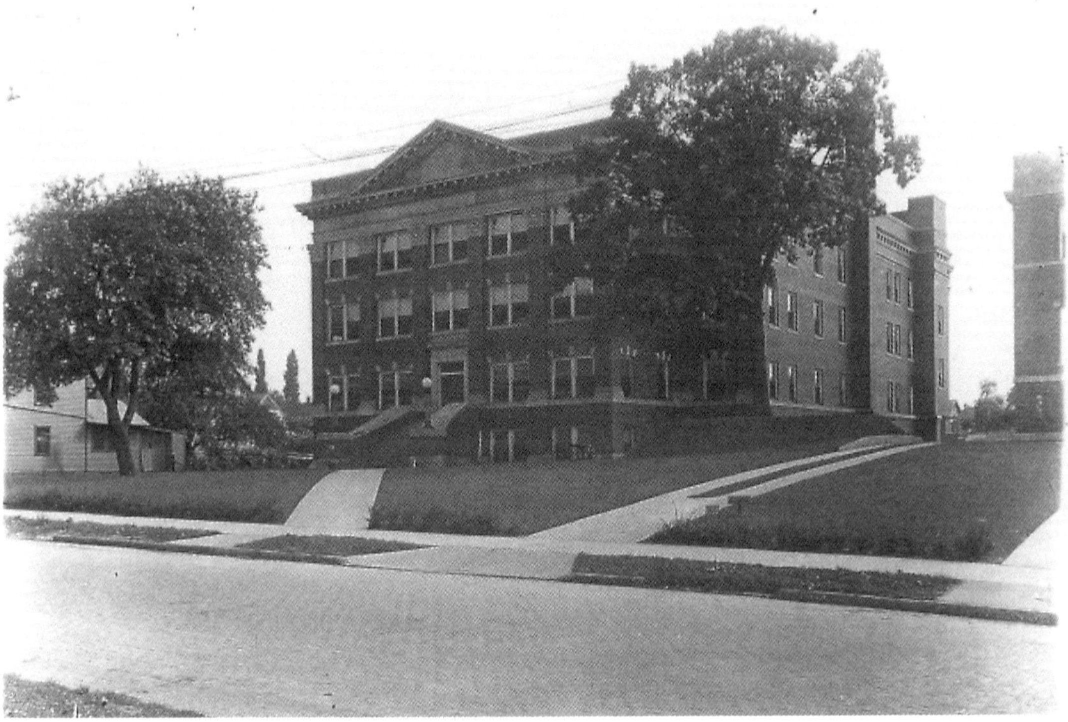

Peoples Hospital, 1916. The Rubber City's new west-side hospital was three stories high, 130 feet long, 80 feet wide, and constructed of brick, tile, and concrete. Total cost: $90,000. **Pockrandt Collection, University of Akron Archives**

tal's sprawling, 30-acre campus.

By the second decade of the 20th century, Akron was booming, as thousands sought jobs in the rubber factories. The rapidly growing town needed another hospital, one located on the west side. According to George Knepper's book, *Akron, City at the Summit*, founders named the hospital "Peoples" because "they wanted the community to feel this new institution was 'theirs.' The People concept was one of good medical care coupled with friendliness and understanding." The 125-bed hospital opened on West Cedar Street in 1915, with a staff of twenty-five, one X-ray machine, one surgical suite, one delivery room, a one-room laboratory, and a small emergency room (whose first patient had fractured his arm cranking his automobile, a harbinger of auto injuries to come).

Department store founder and a leader in Akron's Catholic community, Michael O'Neil (whose son, William, founded General Tire), gave $100,000 to start St. Thomas Hospital, which opened in 1928. Perched on the north rim of Akron's Little Cuyahoga River Valley, St. Thomas Hospital was administered for many years by the Sisters of Charity of Saint Augustine. The hospital's name not only honors Saint Thomas Aquinas, it is an indirect reference to the Reverend Thomas F. Mahar, pastor of Akron's St. Vincent Parish for thirty-four years.

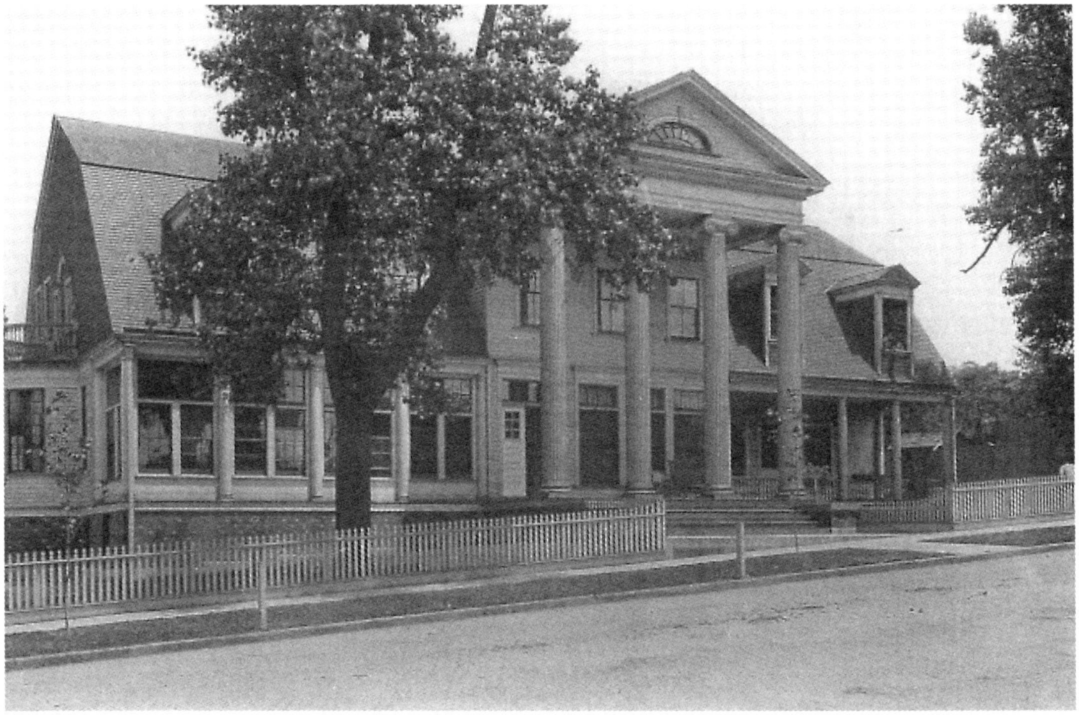

Mary Day Nursery and Children's Hospital, 1898. Akron's first pediatric hospital and its first department of orthopaedic surgery was located on the city's east side on Buchtel Avenue. **University of Akron Archives**

Children's Hospital grew out of the Akron Day Nursery, organized in 1890 to provide child care for working mothers. In 1891, George Todd Perkins donated a house on High Street in honor of the birth of his granddaughter, Mary Perkins Raymond, and the nursery was renamed Mary Day Nursery. In 1905, in cooperation with Akron City Hospital, Mary Day Nursery added the Ward for Crippled Children. This ward served as the pediatric division of City Hospital and, later, Peoples Hospital, until a new Children's Hospital opened in 1928.

Fractured limbs and deformities resulting from congenital diseases have always afflicted the human race. In the seventeenth century, Giovanni Alfonso Borelli, the father of biomechanics (orthopaedic surgery's basic science) studied the movement of the human body and its control by the muscles and developed biomechanical theories. According to Michael J. Askew, Ph.D., Director of the Walter A. Hoyt, Jr., M.D. Musculoskeletal Laboratory, "Further development of Borelli's work had to await three relatively recent technological events: First, Marie Curie's discovery of radium and the subsequent development of x-ray examination of the bony structure of the body by Wilhelm Roentgen in 1895. Second, the Nobel Prize winning work of Archibald Hill on the mechanics of the muscle. Third, the pioneering work of Edward Muybridge who employed photography technology to document the gait pattern of horses. Muybridge wagered that a horse in full gallop had all four hooves off the ground. He won his bet, expanded his study to human motion, founded gait analysis, and was a founder of modern biomechanics."

These discoveries greatly strengthened the musculoskeletal surgeon's armamentarium, which had been sorely limited in the nineteenth century's "strap and buckle" era. Orthopaedics entered the "osteotomy and fusion" era in the twentieth century. Better knowledge of the basic sciences led to technical advances while anesthesia and asepsis contributed to the safety of patients undergoing orthopaedic surgery. The concept of rehabilitation, before and after surgery, so as to restore normal function, took root, grew, and would flower in the Second World War.

American orthopaedics, in transition for the first two decades of the twentieth century, was recognized as a distinct surgical specialty by 1920. Curing the crippling diseases that struck children played a major role in this twenty-year transition period. (The crippled child is at the root of the name "orthopaedics." Nicholas Andre titled his 1741 treatise on deformities in children, *L'Orthopedie*; coining the term by combining two Greek words: orthos, meaning "straight, free from deformity," and pais, "child.") Akron's first orthopaedic clinic opened at Children's Hospital in June, 1918, directed by Walter A. Hoyt, Sr. The clinic's task, according to the *Akron Beacon Journal*, was "reclaiming crippled children...those with crooked spines, perhaps from infantile paralysis, with tuberculosis of the knee, the hip, the spine, hunchbacked and bowlegged children, together with those with club feet...All will be made whole...Pioneers of orthopaedics have established the fact that all of these deformities, whether hereditary or acquired, may be corrected."

The orthopaedic clinic soon showed its worth to the community, tripling in size its first year. Mary Day Nursery had moved across town to Locust Street in 1917, giving Children's more space at 43 Buchtel Avenue. The hospital followed the nursery crosstown in 1928, becoming a near-west-side neighbor of Peoples Hospital. (Dr. Hoyt's daughter, Dorothy, suffering from an infected mastoid, was brought to Children's by ambulance and admitted, the new hospital's first patient, according to her brother, Walter.) Children's quickly grew into a general pediatric hospital. Corrective orthopaedics made up half the hospital's admissions in 1929.

In December 1918, only six months after the orthopaedic clinic opened, Children's physicians established a clinic for poliomyelitis (infantile paralysis) patients. Today, it is difficult to imagine the fear infantile paralysis inspired. For the first half of the twentieth century, however, infantile paralysis, or polio, cast its annual pall over the summer season. As the century lengthened, epidemics worsened. Doctors battled this cyclical, infectious viral disease until the 1950's when development of the Salk and Sabin vaccines virtually eliminated polio in the United States.

Children's orthopaedic department, staffed by Drs. Walter A. Hoyt, Sr., Fowler B. Roberts, and Harold R. Conn, was nationally recognized in the thirties when President Franklin D. Roosevelt, an adult polio victim, used the "bully pulpit" of his office to bring national attention to the disease. Roosevelt's influence led to the formation of the National Foundation for Infantile Paralysis in 1937. Dr. Hoyt, chairman of Children's Hospital Department of Orthopaedic Surgery, accepted an appointment to the Foundation's orthopaedic council at that time. The March of Dimes, held on President Roosevelt's birthday, was the first nationwide drive to fund medical research that, it was hoped, would lead to the elimination of a specific disease.

Another national fund raiser, the President's Birthday Ball, began in January, 1937. According to the *Akron Beacon Journal*, Akronites raised $2,400 that Depression year "for local work among the handicapped, funds [being] distributed 70 percent locally and 30 percent to the national headquarters." The 1938 ball celebrating F.D.R.'s birth struck a sour note, however, when the national organization requested 100 percent of the proceeds. Summit County organizers, with Dr. Hoyt's support, threatened to withdraw from the party unless national plans changed. "I'm in agreement with the foundation's four-point program to wage war on infantile paralysis on a national front," Hoyt said. "But I also agree with (University of Akron) President Simmons and the county committee that a large share of the birthday ball funds should be distributed locally."

Akron's first orthopaedic residency program, established in 1946, has its roots in City Hospital's Department of General Surgery back when the century was young and orthopaedics or "trauma" was a division of that department. Medical practice was not high tech then, nor as extensively regulated as today. Speaking of regulations, William M. Davis, M.D. City/ Children's orthopaedic residency program, class of '53, recalled that his grandfather "practiced medicine two years before he finished medical school! After two years of med school, he and my grandma ran out of money. So, they went down to Berlin, Ohio, Berlin Crossroads. She ran the post office and he practiced medicine." Two years later, the Davises returned to Columbus, he completed his studies at Ohio State and obtained his M.D. degree.

In the teens, twenties, and thirties, a practicing physician interested in sharpening his skills in orthopaedics designed his own postgraduate course. In a talk to the Ohio Orthopaedic Society in 1982, Walter A. Hoyt, Jr., M.D., recalled that his father "came to Akron in 1916 as a general surgeon. He taught himself orthopaedics after coming to Akron, supplemented by a six month period with Arthur Legg and associates in Boston and three months with Michael Hoke in Atlanta, Georgia. He was one of the major instigators and planners of the Crippled Children's program in Ohio, and organized the concept of the specialty of orthopaedics in Akron. His outreach was significant in that he had clinics in Canton, Dover, New Philadelphia, and Alliance."

The doctors who practiced orthopaedics in Akron in the 1920's and 1930's were, like Hoyt, Sr., general surgeons who worked their way toward becoming specialists while in practice and at the same time laid the foundation for the program they would establish after World War II.

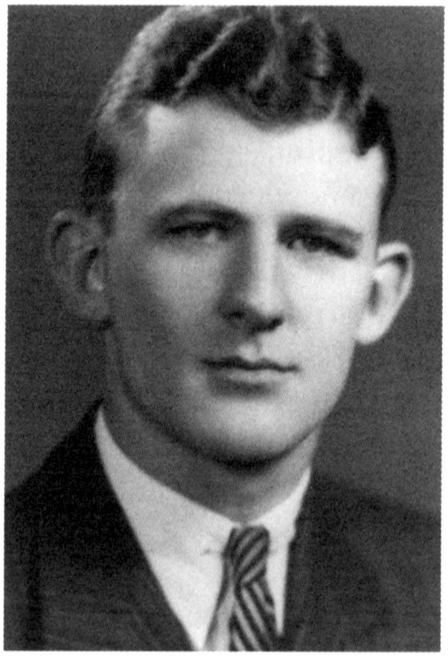

James W. Parks. A second generation teacher, Dr. Parks' curriculum in the 1960s' included implementing the new Medicare law in Summit County.

William A. Parks, M.D., was the first Akron physician to indicate an interest in bone and joint surgery. A graduate of Rush Medical College, William Parks interned at City Hospital in 1909, with a general surgery residency in 1910 and 1911. He practiced orthopaedic and traumatic surgery until his death in 1951. His son, James W. Parks, M.D., shared his father's interest, took a residency at City (class of '49) in orthopaedics, making the Drs. Parks the first father-son team in that specialty at the hospital. A native of Akron, James Parks also served as Chief of Staff at Saint Thomas Hospital. In the sixties, he chaired the Summit County Medical Society's Committee on Contract Medical Practice. In this capacity, James Parks helped implement the new Medicare Law and was honored for his work with a special resolution of commendation.

City's general surgery residency was a two year program in the early years: first year, trauma, second year, general surgery. Carl R. Steinke, M.D., arrived in 1917 and played a significant role in the hospital's surgical training in the twenties and thirties. Steinke was well qualified for the task, having received an excellent postgraduate medical education. A 1909 graduate of the University of Pennsylvania's School of Medicine, he spent six months doing special laboratory work at the Pennsylvania Hospital of Philadelphia, interned at Philadelphia's Episcopal Hospital January 1910 to July 1911, then took a fellowship at the Mayo Clinic.

Steinke recognized the importance of a solid scientific background in medicine. He and H. Vernon Sharp, M.D., developed City's first animal laboratory and its first organized medical library in 1929. Their work paid off, for in 1930, Akron City was one of only seven Ohio hospitals approved by the American Medical Association for surgical training. At a time when most hospitals used indigent clinic patients, Dr. Steinke brought the private patient into the teaching process. He also gave the chief resident more responsibility, allowing the fledgling surgeon to write orders and perform surgery under the watchful eye of the attending physician. Scientific medicine requires research, and Steinke published on a variety of topics relating to orthopaedics - dislocation of the hip, fractures of the femur, spinal tumors, and surgery of the posterior spinal roots.

Fowler B. Roberts, M.D., had been in general practice for several years when he served a preceptorship in orthopaedic surgery under W.A. Hoyt, Sr. from 1927 to 1929. Dr. Roberts was among the first Akron practitioners to attend the University of Pennsylvania Graduate School of Medicine where he earned a Master of Science in orthopaedic surgery. Upon returning to Akron in the depths of the Great Depression, he limited his practice to orthopaedic surgery. Fowler Roberts was a bridge builder, strengthening contacts between Akron General, Children's (where he primarily practiced), and City Hospitals. With Hoyt, Sr, he was a prime mover in City/Children's and General/Children's orthopaedic residency programs. Dr. Roberts' son, James, followed him into orthopaedics.

The surgeons all practiced "bring backs," that is, going to a conference, bringing back a procedure, instrument, or occasionally, even an operating table, to share with their colleagues. Speaking in the sixties of the development of City's orthopaedic program, Edwin L. Mollin, M.D., an early teacher, recalled that "Dr. F.B. Roberts came back from [the University of] Pennsylvania with the Gill osteotome, which may well be the most used instrument in orthopaedic surgery." (When Mollin tried to collect material for his talk, he was "amazed at the paucity of retrievable information." Nevertheless, his informal review of early medical education at City contains valuable snapshots of his colleagues and their work.)

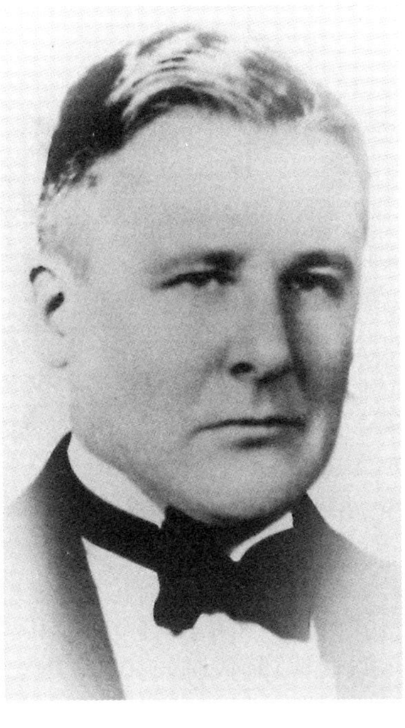

Rey V. Luce: Like his contemporaries, Dr. Luce's practice was not confined to orthopaedics. **Summa Health System**

Modern warfare has had a great impact on orthopaedic surgery's development. Two of Akron's early teachers, Rey V. Luce, M.D., and Harold R. Conn, M.D., served with the British Army Medical Corps in World War I. Later, Conn was chief of the amputation service at Walter Reed Hospital. Luce interned at City in 1913-14 and enlisted in the British Army Medical Corps in 1916. He trained in bone and joint surgery at the Alder Hey Military Orthopaedic Hospital in Liverpool, England, and served a year in Base Hospital #8 in France. Dr. Luce returned to staff in 1919, was elected president of the Summit County Medical Society in 1920, and served as

City's Chief of Staff in 1927 and 1946.

Exposure to British orthopaedists' procedures and techniques in World War I proved valuable to the development of American orthopaedics. One of Rey Luce's teachers at Alder Hey, the charismatic Sir Robert Jones, director of Britain's orthopaedic medical services, greatly influenced these young surgeons who adopted many of the techniques Jones had introduced in the British Army. Furthermore, upon returning home, Americans who had worked with Jones established the Robert Jones Club, whose members met annually to exchange scientific information and, not incidentally, to promote the specialty of orthopaedics in America. Founding Jones Club members included LeRoy Abbott, Carl Badgley, Guy Caldwell, Paul Colonna, Albert Key, and Philip Wilson, each of whom strongly influenced the development of American orthopaedic surgery in the post-First World War years and beyond.

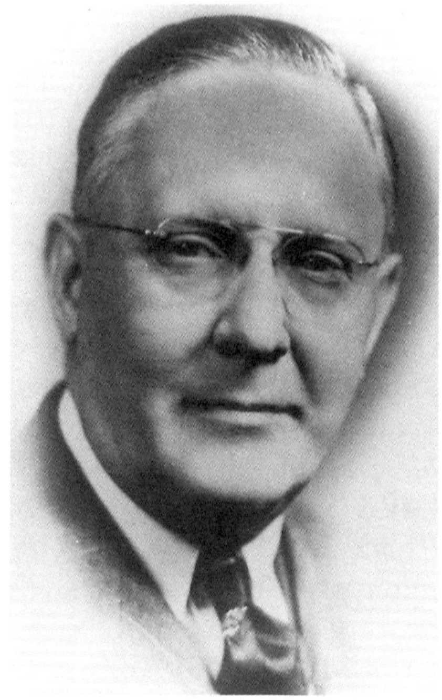

Harold R. Conn: Dr. Conn published eight journal articles and co-authored two textbooks about orthopaedic surgery during his tenure as medical director of all Goodyear Tire and Rubber Company domestic plants. **Summa Health System**

The inspiration for all this, Sir Robert Jones, pioneered in treating war wounds of the extremities A British soldier sustaining an open fracture of the femur in 1914 faced wretched odds, 80 percent chance of dying from shock and sepsis. Jones modified a splint devised in 1875 by his uncle, bone-setter-surgeon Hugh Owen Thomas, to treat tuberculosis of the knee and fractures of the femur. Jones's modified Thomas splint limited local blood loss into the extremity by tightening the fascial envelope and by using local pressure to restrict bleeding. Military surgeons began using the modified Thomas splint in 1915. By 1917, death from fractures of the femur had been reduced to less than 16 percent.

A specialist in industrial trauma, Harold Conn came to Akron in 1920 to head the Goodyear Tire and Rubber Company's ten-bed hospital. Edwin Mollin recalled him as "a hard driving orthopaedist who developed the concept of a traumatic service apart from general surgery....writing papers was not a big feature of Akron's clinical medicine in the thirties, but Dr. Conn wrote on fractures of the os calcis." Conn also developed an apparatus for reduction of os calcis fractures, an industrial injury which had a unique twist at Goodyear, given its lighter-than-air program. A worker sliding down an airship's shroud line would sometimes be forced to let go when friction burned

Though heel bone breaks incurred constructing airships are long past, deer hunting season can bring a rash of such fractures according to Ian Alexander, M.D., subspecialist in foot and ankle. "You know how hunters go up in tree stands to hunt deer? Sometimes they fall out of them, land on their heels and break their heels. They fall ten, fifteen feet, commonly break their heels and nothing else."

his hands and he lost his grip. The man usually landed feet first on the cement floor, often fracturing both heel bones.

Dr. Conn developed several other orthopaedic appliances including, in 1944, the pneumatic tourniquet used in extremity surgery to prevent intra-operative hemorrhage. Perhaps his best known monograph is *The Battalion Medical Officer*, which was distributed to all medical officers in the U.S. military in the Second World War. And, according to Dr. Mollin, Conn could improvise. Mollin recalled his own intern days "when a patient came in with a fracture of the femoral shaft, a huge man....Dr. Conn went over to the engineering or maintenance area and made a Thomas splint with the ring diameter of 36 inches."

Adrian E. Davis, M.D., interned at City Hospital in 1926 and proved a good source, and subject, for Edwin Mollin's 1960's review of orthopaedics at City. Davis completed his surgical residency in 1929 and later went to Boston for further training in orthopaedics with A.E. Codman. Dr. Davis introduced the technique of stabilizing a subtrochanteric osteotomy with a reversed Blount blade plate. A Fellow of the American College of Surgeons, Davis succeeded W.A. Hoyt, Sr., as head of the orthopaedic service and head of the orthopaedic residency program in 1949. He served in that capacity through 1961 when he was succeeded by Walter A. Hoyt, Jr., M.D.

Mollin said Davis "nailed the first hip at City Hospital. He had a patient with a basilar neck fracture; this was at the time that Smith-Peterson was developing the tri-flanged nail. Dr. Davis had Mr. Greenbaum, a brace man from Cleveland — orthotics not yet on the scene — make for him four threaded wires, or pins. A closed reduction and internal fixation using these threaded pins was accomplished. The position held and the fracture healed. Another doctor obtained similar pins, but used them on a sub-capital fracture. Unfortunately, the metal was straight from Main Street Hardware — the nails rusted — broke — and the fracture collapsed, requiring a second operation."

While writing papers was, as Mollin said, "not a big feature of Akron's clinical medicine in the thirties," some local clinicians, A.E. Davis, Carl Steinke, and Harold Conn, to name only three, did do research; it helped them in their work. Perhaps Dr. Davis's crowning achievement came in co-authoring, with Drs. W.A. Hoyt, Sr. and George Van Buren, a paper on the "Use of Sulfathiazole in the treatment of osteomyelitis." Hoyt, Sr. presented the paper at the American Medical Association meeting in Cleveland, Ohio, June 5, 1941. Later, the paper won the Gold Medal at the annual meeting of the American Academy of Orthopaedic Surgeons [A.A.O.S.]. The Davis, Hoyt, Sr., Van Buren paper was mentioned in the *New England Journal of Medicine* as recently as February 11, 1993 in "Case Records of the Massachusetts General Hospital."

Orr's closed plaster technique was still employed to treat osteomyelitis when W.A. Hoyt, Jr. was an orthopaedic surgery resident at the Shrine Hospital in Greeneville, South Carolina in the mid-forties. A boy with osteomyelitis in the femur presented on a steamy Sunday morning. "He was scheduled to have his cast removed," Hoyt recalled years later, "have the dressings changed, and a new cast applied on Monday morning. So, in preparation for that, I bi-valved the cast, took the top half off. It was a hot summer day and, as I took off the cast, the maggots began to hatch and there were thousands of flies in the operating room. In the old days, we used maggots in cleaning wounds, but these just came from the child's home environment."

The discovery of antibiotics in the thirties greatly expanded the physician's armamentarium, sometimes eliminating surgical intervention. Sulfathiazole, for example, made possible the non-operative treatment of osteomyelitis, an infection in bone that was a major cause of disability in children. Before sulfathiazole, the treatment of choice for osteomyelitis was the "closed plaster technique," a procedure that came out of World War I. In this procedure, developed by Dr. Winnett Orr to treat open fractures (a common battlefield injury), the surgeon thoroughly debrided the wound, packed it with petrolatum gauze, and immobilized the extremity in a plaster-of-paris cast.

The younger members of the first generation, Beyer, Birnbaum, Bischoff, Doran, Minnig, and Mollin, arrived in the thirties, the era of the Great Depression. According to the *Akron Beacon Journal*, "Akron's industrial unemployment rate hit a staggering 60 percent in 1932. The national economy, with unemployment of 23.6 percent, looked robust by comparison."

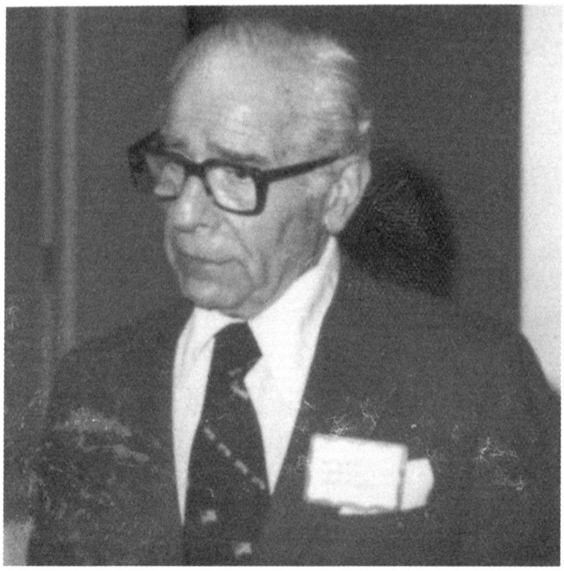

Millard C. Beyer: Dr. Beyer's efforts to upgrade ambulance equipment and certify ambulance personnel in advanced first aid led to passage, in 1955, of Akron's first ordinance regulating ambulance companies. **Department of Orthopaedics, Summa Health System**

Millard C. Beyer, M.D., interned at City Hospital 1929-30, served as medical resident in 1931-

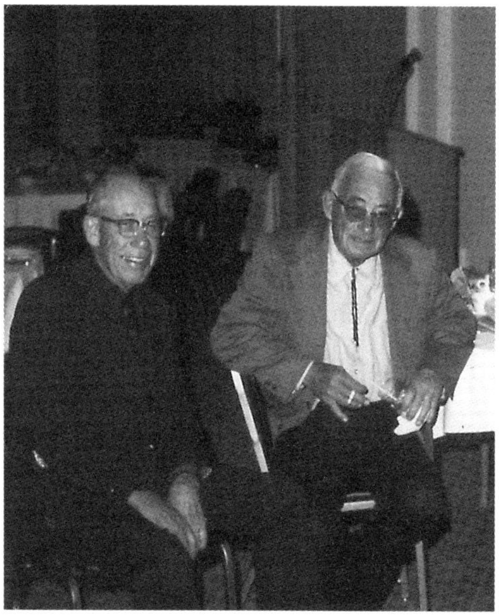

Hoyt Society Resident's Conference, 1978, from left to right: George H. Bischoff and Adrian E. Davis.
Summa Health System

32, surgical resident in 1932-33, chief resident in surgery, 1933-34, and was granted junior staff privileges in orthopaedic and traumatic surgery in 1935. Dr. Beyer presided over the Summit County Medical Society in 1953 and helped organize the county's emergency medical program. The Harriman Award for Distinguished Volunteer Service, highest award bestowed by the American Red Cross, is one of Dr. Beyer's honors.

I.R. Birnbaum, M.D., interned at City Hospital 1929-30, served one and a half years' residency in general surgery, and one and a half years in orthopaedics. Dr. Birnbaum was appointed to the junior staff in orthopaedic surgery in 1933.

George Bischoff, M.D., paid his way to medical school at Northwestern University by shepherding a train load of sheep from Salt Lake City to Chicago. He interned at City in 1935-36, then served a two year residency in general surgery at City and Children's. Dr. Bischoff directed Idaho's State Crippled Children's Services for two and a half years. After five years in the army, he returned to Akron and completed his last year of training as senior resident in orthopaedics, 1946-47.

Patrick C. Doran, M.D., was born in Akron, graduated from St. Vincent's High School, received his Bachelor of Arts degree from Notre Dame and his medical degree from Western Reserve University. He interned at City Hospital 1930-31, then went to Children's Hospital in orthopaedics in 1930-31 and St. Thomas Hospital in 1931-32. He served as City's chief of staff in 1956.

Donald I. Minnig, M.D., served an internship at City Hospital in 1938-39, then served a residency and fellowship in orthopaedic surgery at the Cleveland Clinic from 1939 to 1941. Dennis S. Weiner, M.D.,

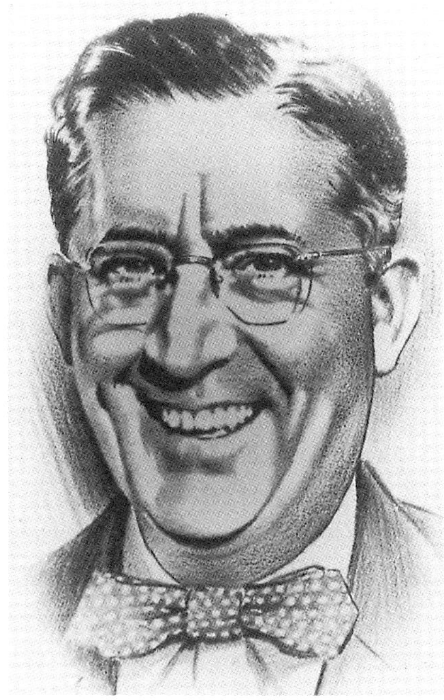

Patrick C. Doran: Akron born, Dr. Doran served as Chief of Staff at St. Thomas and Children's Hospitals and was Chief of Staff at City Hospital from May 1956 until his death in March 1957.
Summa Health System

chairman of Children's Department of Orthopaedic Surgery, recalls that Dr. Minnig also trained in Missouri with Dr. MacBride, an innovator in bunion surgery. Dr. Minnig practiced primarily at Children's, Akron General, and Barberton Hospitals. He served as president of the Summit County Medical Society in 1959 and president of the Ohio Orthopaedic Society in 1963.

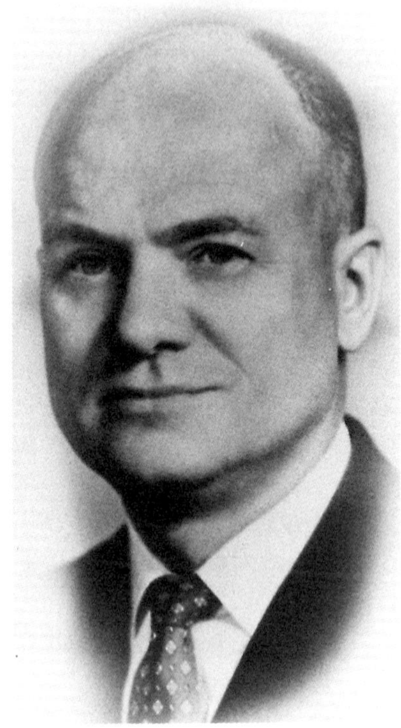

Edwin L. Mollin: Dr. Mollin served as Chief of Staff of Akron City Hospital in 1962 and also donated hundreds of hours as an adviser to Ohio's Bureau of Crippled Children's Services.
Summa Health System

Edwin L. Mollin interned at City Hospital in 1937, served one year of residency under Dr. Hoyt, Sr., then was a resident in orthopaedic surgery at the University of Michigan, 1939-42 under Dr. Carl Badgley. He returned to Akron after World War II and joined Dr. Hoyt, Sr., his father-in-law, in the practice of orthopaedic surgery. Together, they founded outpatient clinics throughout northeastern Ohio under the auspices of the Bureau of Crippled Children (now the Bureau of Maternal and Child Health).

Dennis Weiner remembers Edwin Mollin as "a hard working, inexhaustible, industrious physician." In August 1984, the Ohio State Senate passed a resolution praising Mollin for his work with crippled children. He conducted more than one thousand orthopaedic field clinics during his forty-year association with the Bureau of Crippled Children and served for thirty-six years on its medical advisory committee. He was a member of the Board of Counselors for the American Academy of Orthopaedic Surgeons and served as president of the Ohio Orthopaedic Society, president of the Summit County Medical Society, and chief of staff at Akron City Hospital.

As staff members in one of seven AMA-certified teaching hospitals in Ohio, City's clinicians worked hard to maintain their surgical residency accreditation. In the mid-1930's the American College of Surgeons accredited a cancer clinic at Akron City Hospital (one of only four in the State of Ohio). Chief of Surgery, Carl Steinke, brought F.T.(Ted) Moore, M.D. from the University of Michigan to direct City's X-ray and Radium service. A member of the first class to be certified in radiology, Moore received his Radiology Boards in 1935. Edwin Mollin was a surgery resident at the hospital in 1938 and, in his 1960's review of orthopaedics at City, reported that "all [medical] services (reflected) the increased needs or requirements to deliver appropriate health care. Radiology, [with its board-certified chief], was among the services requested to hold teaching clinics. A rotation through pathology was also under consideration. Dr. Robert Allison requested that some gynecology patients be assigned to private staff surgery to improve the educational value of that residency service."

This determination to strengthen City's residency programs reflects important national developments: the founding of the American Academy of Orthopaedic Surgeons and the establishment of its quality control sibling, the American Board of Orthopaedic Surgery. Interest in the specialty had grown since the First World War when returning medical officers founded The Robert Jones Club in order to discuss scientific developments in orthopaedics and promote the specialty among their peers.

So successfully did these Robert Jones Club members generate interest in orthopaedics that, in 1931, nearly four times the expected number of attendees swamped the annual meeting of the venerable American Orthopaedic Association. Founded in 1887, the AOA focuses on academic medicine; prospective members submit scientific papers as part of their initiation into the "by invitation only" organization. This, the specialty's oldest professional society, simply could not accommodate the rapid influx, nor did it wish to. Orthopaedics needed a more inclusive professional society, one that could accommodate everyone.

> If you expect sixty for dinner and 225 show up, that strains the budget. According to the Academy's history, *1933-1983, Fifty Years of Progress*, "it was customary for the AOA's President to provide entertainment at his own expense for all persons attending the Annual Meeting. This expensive custom was said to be a major reason for organizing the AAOS."

The American Academy of Orthopaedic Surgeons, founded in 1933, provided the best forum for the dissemination of scientific education. The AAOS encourages continuing education, provides access to educational resources, and gives all orthopaedic surgeons a national forum for discussion and scientific interchange. From 1934 on, orthopaedists were admitted to membership by successfully completing part two of the certifying examination.

> The Academy has always welcomed young orthopaedists. Dr. Hoyt, Sr. began the policy of having the senior resident attend the AAOS's annual meeting, his expenses paid by assessing City's senior and junior staff. Only once has there been cause to regret this policy. That occurred when an early resident's champagne tastes overwhelmed his sense of fiscal responsibility. It never happened again.

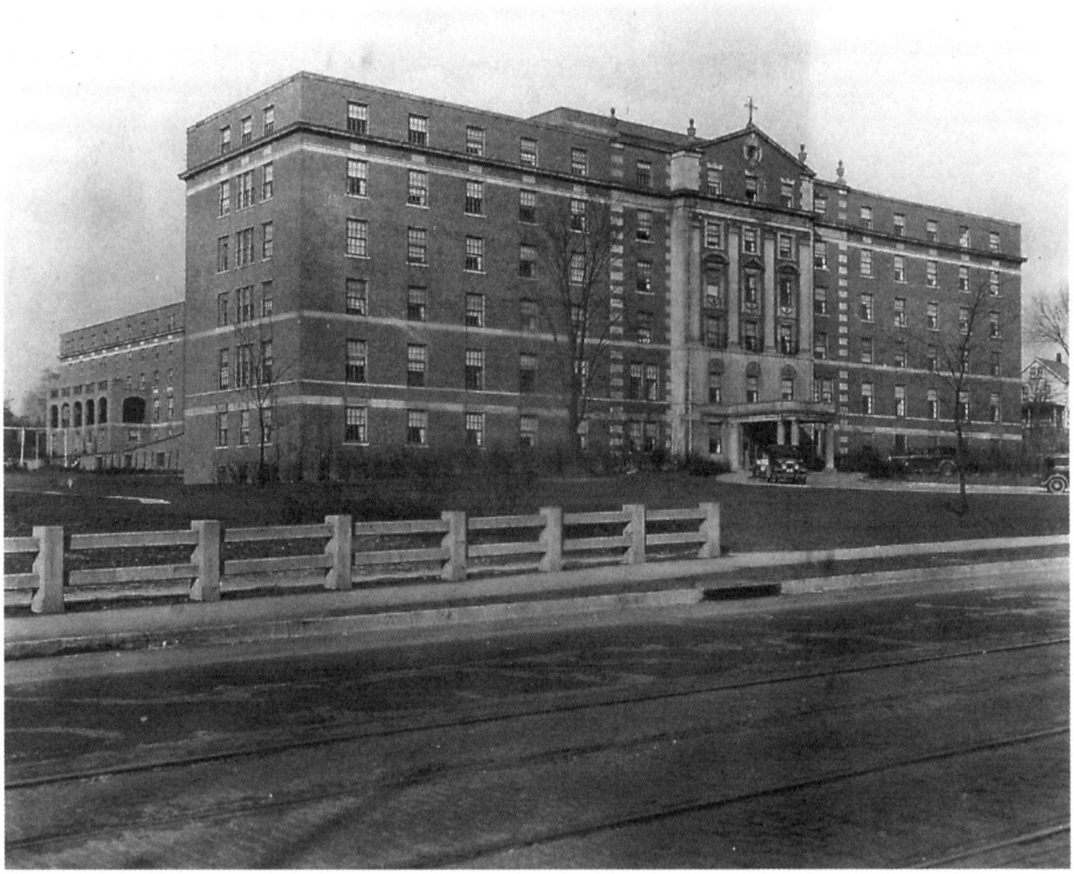

St. Thomas Hospital, 1930. Several early teachers, Bischoff, Conn, Doran, and Hoyt, Sr. among them, had privileges at this north side general hospital. **Pockrandt Collection, University of Akron Archives**

Formal residency education in orthopaedics began at a few medical schools in the mid-thirties. Residents (then called "trainees") served an apprenticeship: "learning by practical experience under skilled workers," just as a nineteenth century medical student apprenticed himself to a "respectable practitioner" for clinical training. Trainees worked with a well-known orthopaedic surgeon who provided a patient population and the opportunity to learn the techniques of surgical management by assisting him in the operating room.

Instruction in the fledgling residencies lacked uniformity, however. In 1934, the American Orthopaedic Association and the American Academy of Orthopaedic Surgeons, together with the American Medical Association, set educational standards and created the American Board of Orthopaedic Surgery to insure those standards were met. Speaking in the 1990's of those early days, W.A. Hoyt, Jr. recalled that "the ABOS insisted that the residencies have a three year time frame. During this three year period, residents had to spend stipulated periods of time in trauma, in adult orthopaedics, in pediatric orthopaedics, in basic science. An individual had to have all that to sit for his certification exam." In 1938, Akron City Hospital's senior staff in general and

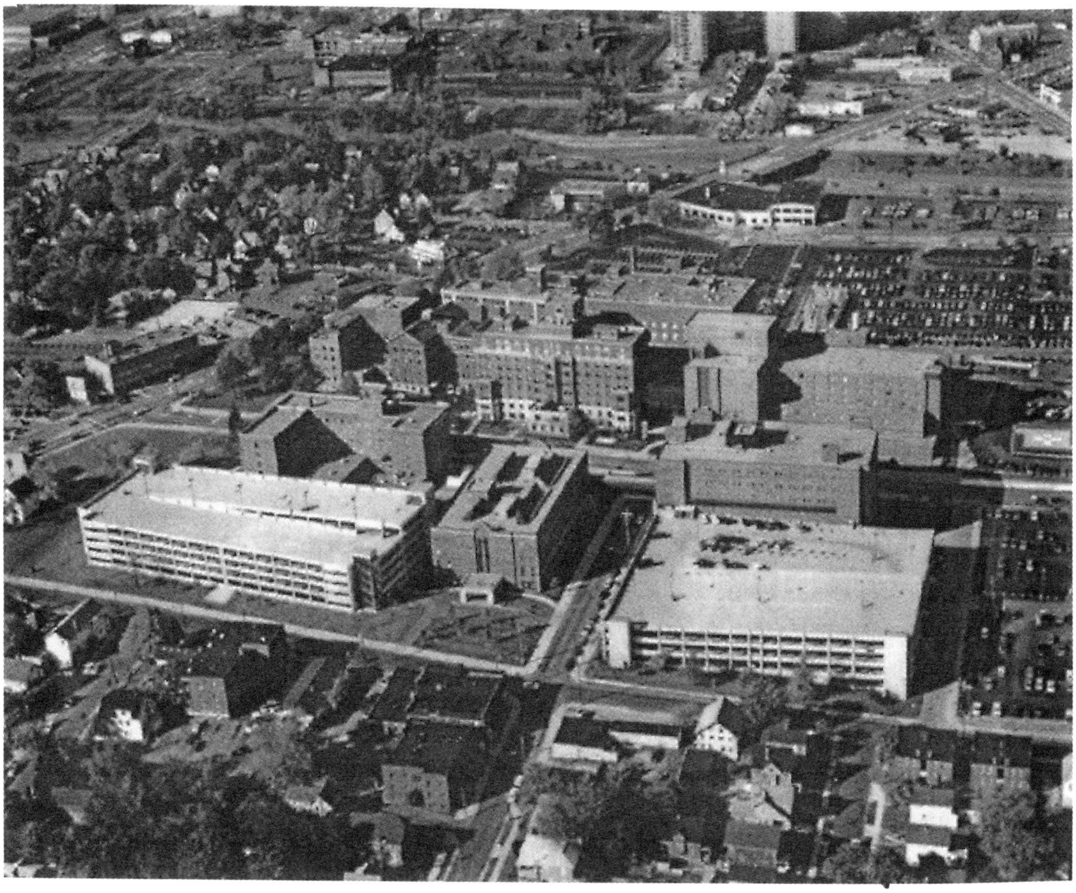

Akron City Hospital today. Typical of the automobile age, two of the largest buildings on City's 30 acre campus are the parking decks in the foreground. **Summa Health System**

trauma surgery followed the national trend and increased the length of their general surgery residency program from two to three years.

World War II - Orthopaedics Comes of Age

The specialty of orthopaedic surgery, born in the First World War, came of age in World War II, a cataclysm that split the twentieth century into two eras - - before and after the most destructive war in history. Prior to the war, most musculoskeletal injuries usually were treated by general surgeons. Most of Akron's early teachers trained as general surgeons, and then, on their own initiative, studied with orthopaedic specialists after they were in practice. W.A. Hoyt, Sr., for example, did all types of surgery, including brain surgery, just as his teacher, C. B. Nancrede, had done. After the war, with accreditation and certification firmly in place, treating musculoskeletal injuries slowly became the province of the board certified orthopaedic surgeon.

The specialty of orthopaedics came of age during the Second World War and so did a new generation of physicians who, through their wartime experiences, were eager to study and practice the specialty. One of this generation, Charles H. Herndon, M.D., spent his career "up the road," so to speak, in Cleveland, Ohio. He joined the faculty of Western Reserve University School of Medicine in 1949 as the first full-time orthopaedist in that institution's history. Herndon was an intern at Cleveland's University Hospitals in 1941 when he heard Philip D. Wilson, a charter member of The Robert Jones Club, speak about the American Hospital in Oxford, England. Following the Battle of Britain, Wilson collected funds and recruited young surgeons to go to England. Persuaded by Wilson's appeal, Herndon received permission to join the unit and sailed for England in January 1942.

Forty years later, at the close of a distinguished career, Herndon recalled his tour at the American Hospital, which became the Second General Hospital when American troops arrived in August 1942. There were the English orthopaedists "who had a strong influence on the management of war wounds in the allied forces." There were Americans such as Frank Stinchfield, "who established in Coventry the first rehabilitation unit in the American armed forces. At the same time, Howard Rusk was beginning to develop rehabilitation units in the zone of the interior...Rusk became known for his work in rehabilitation and ultimately, as Director of New York Hospital, established the specialty of physiatry [physical medicine]."

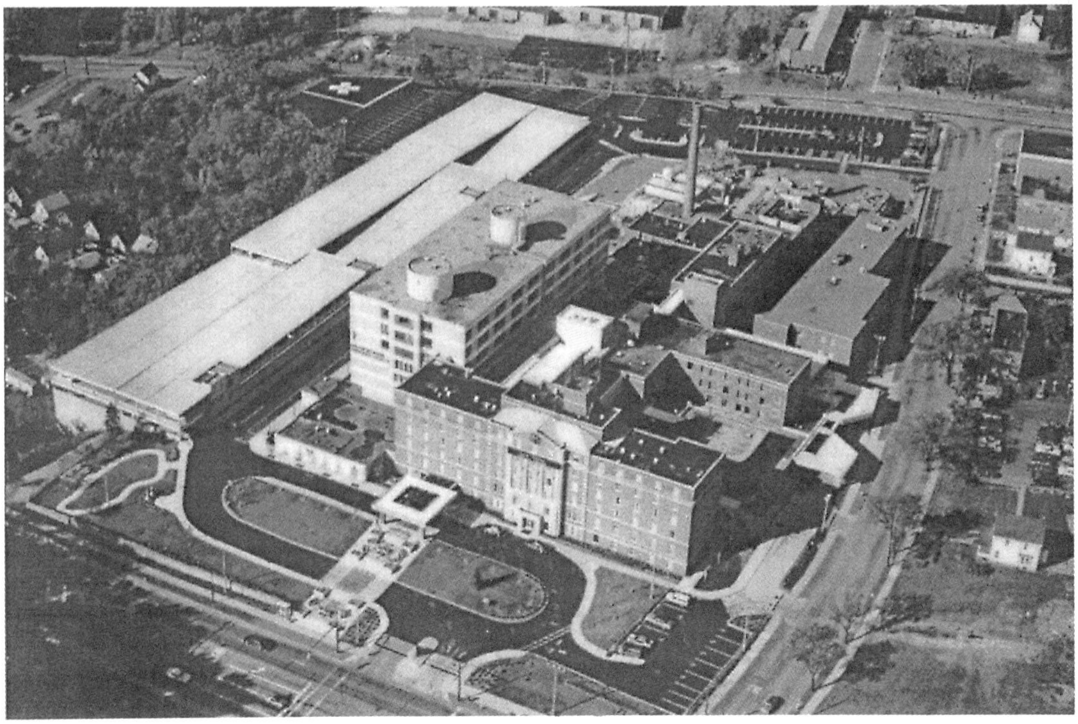

St. Thomas Hospital today. Now part of Summa Health System, St. Thomas sprawls across an entire block. **Summa Health System**

The war gave orthopaedists, as Herndon later said, "tremendous experience in the use of plaster and [in the] conservative management of extremity injuries." Indeed, the volume of musculoskeletal injuries in the Second World War was so great that medical corps officers found themselves working as orthopaedic surgeons regardless of their background in civilian practice. Regulations quickly came in place to protect casualties from inexperienced radical surgical management. Open reduction and internal fixation of closed fractures was not permitted. All compound wounds were left open. Forward echelon physicians extensively debrided wounds, treated them with penicillin, which doctors called "The Arthur Fleming Miracle," and immobilized the extremity in plaster. Then the soldier was flown to a general hospital where, as Walter A. Hoyt, Jr. recalled, "more experienced orthopaedists were responsible for secondarily closing these wounds."

Several Akron orthopaedists served in the Second World War. Patrick Doran worked with Mather Cleveland, M.D., the Director of Orthopaedics in the European Theater of Operations. James W. Parks was a medical officer on an aircraft carrier, the USS *San Jacinto*. Millard Beyer spent seventeen months overseas in North Africa and Italy and was decorated for heroism. During one campaign, Dr. Beyer collapsed after working five days and five nights without

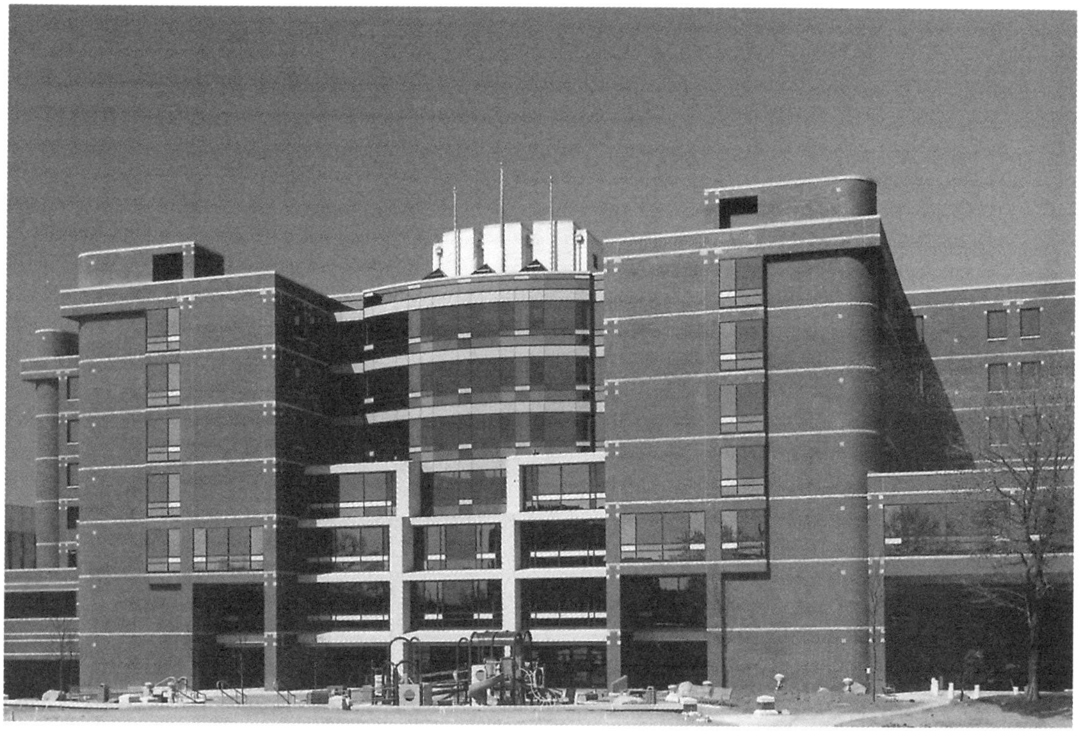

Children's Hospital Medical Center of Akron today. Shown here, Children's new main entrance, which occupies Perkins Square Park, Akron's original Public Square. Now among the ten largest pediatric hospitals in the nation, Children's began as a day care center, added a Ward for Crippled Children in 1905, and, in 1916, established Northeastern Ohio's first Department of Orthopaedics.

Children's Hospital Medical Center

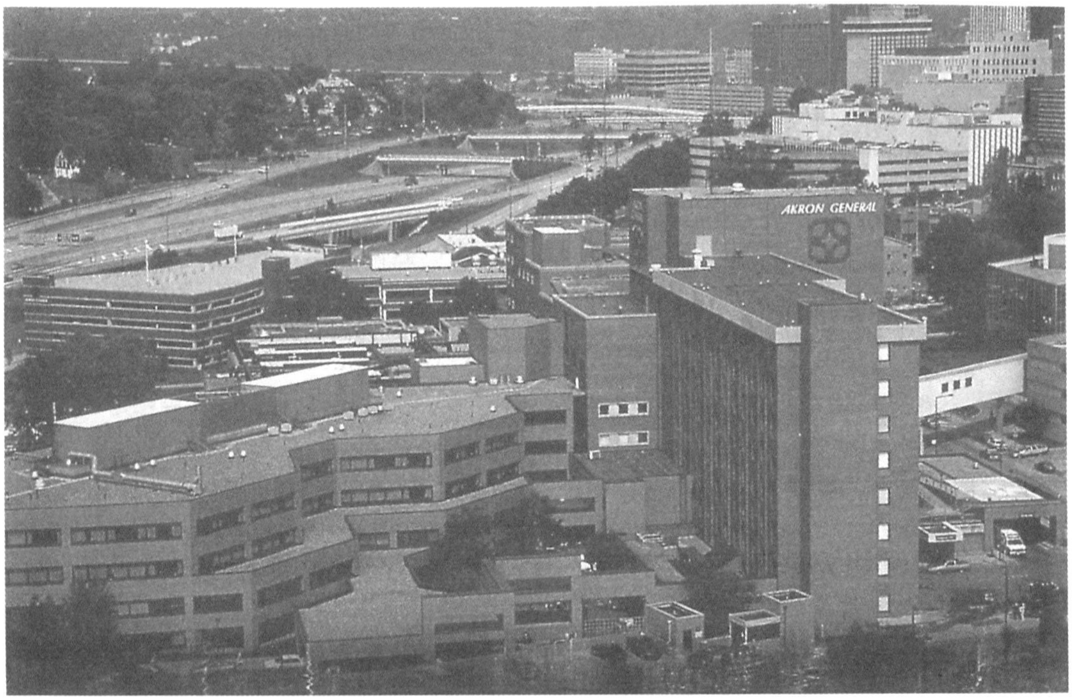

Akron General Medical Center today. Peoples Hospital "three stories high, 130 feet long and 80 feet wide," has long since disappeared into this modern medical complex. **Akron General Medical Center**

sleep or relief. George Bischoff served five years in the army, four of which were in orthopaedic and trauma services at station, general, and evacuation hospitals. A.E. Davis served at the Oakland Naval Hospital and spent eighteen months at sea aboard the USS *Relief* in the Pacific. Edwin Mollin served as an orthopaedic surgeon at the 17th General Army Hospital in Naples, Italy. Don Minnig was chief of orthopaedic surgery at Camp Shelby, Mississippi and at the 133rd General Hospital in the Philippines. W.A. Hoyt, Jr. served with George Patton's Third Army in an evacuation hospital from Omaha Beach to Austria. He performed two thousand operations in nine months and was awarded the Bronze Star by General Patton.

Conservative care paid off. Wound management in World War II was very successful; primary healing after delayed closure was over 90 percent. Big challenges remained, however. Recalling those days, Dr. Hoyt said that "areas such as fracture immobilization (Küntscher's Rod), internal and external skeletal transfixion, hand surgery, amputation surgery, and prosthetics showed the need for technological developments and biomechanical research." And he recalled a night at his evacuation hospital "when Army Rangers got into an electrically controlled mine field and we had fifty young men with amputations come into our unit in a matter of a couple of hours."

(That was only one night, in one unit, during the war.) "Those Rangers (and hundreds like them) required expert prosthetic care," Hoyt said. "This need stimulated the development of prosthetic centers around the country after the war."

Under the direction of Major General Norman T. Kirk, Surgeon General of the Army and the first Medical Corps officer to specialize in orthopaedic surgery, the U.S. Army established prosthetic units and hand surgery units in each service command. Kirk staffed these units with talented specialists who passed along their knowledge and expertise to scores of physicians. One instructor, Clinton Compere, was a prosthetics expert who later developed the Rehabilitation Institute of Chicago. Another, hand surgeon Sterling Bunnell, served as a civilian consultant for two years during the war and taught many medical officers surgery of the hand.

World War II created a tremendous demand for orthopaedic surgeons, a demand that continued unabated in military hospitals long after the shooting stopped. William M. Davis's experience illustrates how short was the supply of orthopaedists in 1946. A graduate of the Army Specialist Training Program at Ohio State's Medical School, Davis owed the military two years service. W.A. Hoyt, Sr. gave him three months at the end of his internship in 1947 "as a supernumerary resident, which ended in July. By November," Davis continued, "I was chief of orthopaedics at a 750 -bed station hospital at Fort Ord, California - on the basis of three months training. I did approximately two hundred major procedures in two years in the army and when I returned to Akron as a resident, surgery was no mystery to me."

Correctly anticipating a tremendous demand for more residency programs, the American Orthopaedic Association and the American Academy of Orthopaedic Surgeons appointed a Joint Committee on Postgraduate Training late in the war. W.A. Hoyt, Jr. would recall years later that its task was twofold: "It reviewed existing orthopaedic residency programs to assure their quality and it determined the potential of other hospital-based orthopaedic services [such as City's] to provide orthopaedic training. The purpose," Hoyt concluded, "was to increase the capacity to meet the demand for additional residency programs."

Certifying a new program would not be easy, however. The American Medical Association's Council on Graduate Medical Education, determined to maintain program quality over sheer numbers of programs, had already raised the cross bar in preparation for this postwar race to launch new residencies. They had strengthened accreditation requirements, set a January 1946 deadline for all senior staff in an accredited teaching hospital to be board certified in their specialty, and insisted that all residency programs meet board requirements.

On October 29, 1945, W.A. Hoyt, Sr. reviewed for City's staff the AMA rules: First, all residencies should be lengthened to meet board requirements. (City's general surgery staff had complied in 1938.) Second, only board-eligible individuals should be appointed to the junior staff. Third, those junior staff members who had no chance of advancement were to be dropped. Four, so as not to become inbred, they should also appoint doctors to staff who had trained at other hospitals. Five, requirements should be increased for physicians seeking major surgical privileges. Six, the respective service must be consulted when appointing residents to that service. Seven, it was strongly recommended that a department of physical medicine be developed.

Then Dr. Hoyt presented the concept of a combined program at Children's and City Hospitals, stressing that there was an abundant patient population and, though each could act separately for accreditation, joint action would create a stronger proposal. The hospitals did act jointly and, in 1946, the AMA and the American Board of Orthopaedic Surgery provisionally approved Akron's first residency program in orthopaedic surgery. A representative of the AMA's Residency Review Committee, Hugh Smith, M.D., reviewed City/Children's orthopaedic residency program in 1947 and granted full certification.

In the thirty years since Walter Asahel Hoyt, Sr. had arrived in Akron to develop the Rubber City's first Department of Orthopaedic Surgery, graduate medical education had grown steadily. After World War II, it expanded exponentially. Before the war, three-fourths of American physicians described themselves as general practitioners, part-time specialists, or physician/surgeons. After the war, board certification in any of a dozen specialties was essential to being on staff in a teaching hospital. Akron's early teachers trained as general surgeons and, once in practice, became interested in orthopaedics and learned on their own. The succeeding generation would take accredited residencies in orthopaedics and be board certified. Judged by the standards of a major university's medical center, City/Children's residency in orthopaedic surgery was modest. Hoyt, Sr., F.B. Roberts, A.E. Davis, and the others saw the program simply as a continuation of what they had been doing since 1930, educating physicians at a certified teaching hospital.

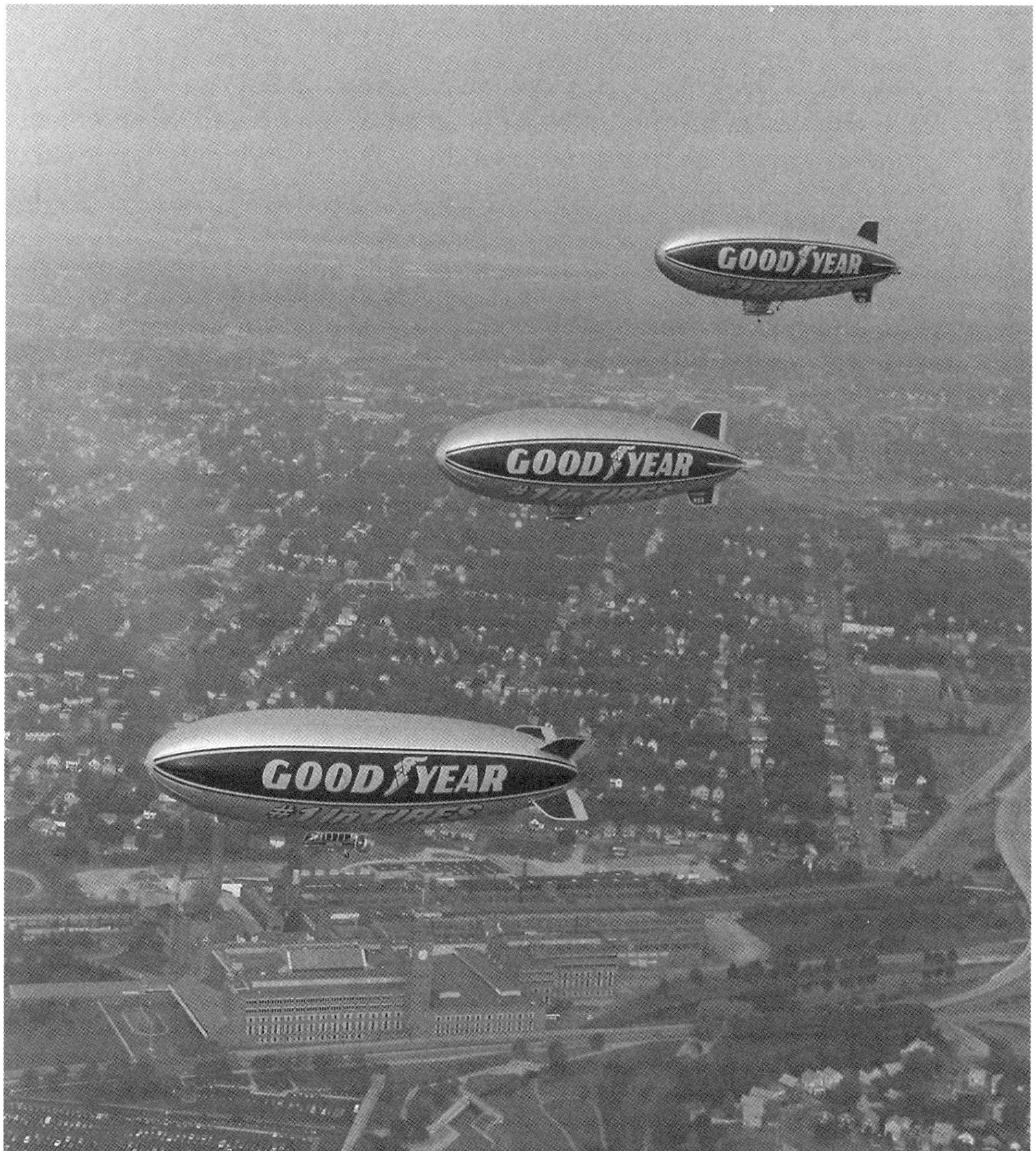

Goodyear blimps fly over Akron. Today, these jolly, blue and gold lighter-than-airships make people smile, but, in the 1947 polio epidemic, their illuminated HEADLINE signs flashed the "new cases" count to Akronites.

Courtesy of The Goodyear Tire and Rubber Company

Chapter Two

1946-1969, Setting the Foundation

Graduate education prospered in the quarter century following World War II, as knowledge in all fields expanded tremendously. The nation's top medical centers engaged in sophisticated research and developed the whole science of orthopaedic surgery. Government agencies and private charities, such as the National Foundation for Infantile Paralysis, financially supported education and research. Orthopaedics' first subspecialty, hand surgery, born in the U.S. Army's wartime hand centers, was officially recognized in 1946 when Sterling Bunnell founded the American Society for Surgery of the Hand. In Akron, two generations of clinicans set the foundation for City/Children's orthopaedic residency and Akron General/Children's program. Leaders in this occasionally daunting task include Adrian E. Davis, Walter A. Hoyt (senior and junior), Donald I. Minnig, Edwin Mollin, Harry O'Dell, and Fowler B. Roberts.

When City/Children's residency in orthopaedic surgery began in 1946, Akron's tire factories were running around the clock and the Rubber City's citizens were prospering after years of depressed economic conditions and wartime shortages. Shoppers crowded Main Street's, multistoried department stores. Downtown bustled, even after dark. People dined at the Garden Grille, Kaase's, Clarks, or, for a special occasion, the elegant Mayflower, the city's premiere hotel. After dinner, they could take in a movie at one of the vast picture palaces along Main Street. Business still boomed when Akron General (formerly Peoples) Hospital's orthopaedic surgery residency began in 1957, but suburban living was taking over. Shopping patterns changed as "malls" evolved, television shuttered Main Street's ornate movie houses, and fewer people ventured downtown after dark.

Early Days

Akron's orthopaedic residencies faced a serious stumbling block until the seventies: no medical school affiliation. The Rubber City's industrial base provided patients by the ton, but nary an ounce of academics. Professors of medicine, secure in their great medical centers, did not believe it possible for students to receive a strong graduate education in a preceptorial setting located in a mill town. W.A. Hoyt, Jr. recalls that from the moment City/Children's program began, "people said, now wait a minute, there's no medical school in Akron. All you have is a bunch of well-trained, aggressive orthopaedic sur-

> The Rubber City's factories ran four six-hour shifts daily in the fifties and sixties. Business boomed and so did industrial accidents. Most manufacturers, railroads, and government services designated certain physicians to care for their injured employees. Harold Conn was physician in charge at Goodyear, which had its own fully equipped hospital then, complete with operating room and ten beds for inpatient care. The Hoyt office served B.F. Goodrich, Columbia Chemical, and Pittsburgh Plate Glass. A.E. Davis captured most of the work from Firestone, the City of Akron, Ohio Edison, and East Ohio Gas, plus some Goodyear referrals. Fowler B. Roberts was attending physician for American Hard Rubber and a general surgeon, Earl Simendinger, directed medical services at General Tire.

geons who are going to teach these residents. Where'll they get basic science?"

Dr. Hoyt chaired City's and Children's departments of orthopaedic surgery for twenty years. A member of the Association of Orthopaedic Chairmen, Hoyt often found himself "on a hot seat over the question of whether an orthopaedic department should be connected with an academic institution. Akron's were not." He defended the non-academic institutions to academe's cream who thought orthopaedic residents in community hospitals got a skim milk education. "We actually debated the merits of having residency programs (such as Akron's) in a non-academic setting," Dr. Hoyt said. His opponents included orthopaedic department chairmen from Harvard, Columbia, and the University of Pennsylvania.

Walter A. Hoyt, Jr. received his B.A. at Amherst College in 1937, earned his M.D. in 1941 at Western Reserve University's School of Medicine, and interned at University Hospital in Cleveland in 1943. He served with Patton's Army in an evacuation hospital in the European Theater. After the war, he took his residency at Duke University and came to Akron in 1949, shortly after his father's untimely death at age 61.

Duke's program exemplified the educational benefits available at the nation's top medical centers. Twenty-five residents, all supported by a grant from the National Foundation for Infantile Paralysis, were the first to participate in Lenox Baker's innovative multi-center residency program. Hoyt considers his Duke residency "a unique opportunity because of the medical centers involved. They included Warm Springs, Georgia, Greenville, South Carolina, the General Hospital at Charlotte, North Carolina, with Oscar Miller, the North Carolina Orthopaedic Children's Hospital under Bill Roberts, and the Alfred I. DuPont Crippled Children's Hospital in Wilmington, Delaware, with Al Shands, as well as the Duke Medical Center with Lenox Baker. Most of the residents arriving on the scene in 1946 had considerable surgical experience in war time. Hence, the speed of learning was enhanced."

Drs. Hoyt, Sr. and Fowler B. Roberts responded to criticism over

Orthopaedics was a division of City's Department of General Surgery in the forties, fifties and sixties. See diagram:

1st year
internship

2nd year
general surgery

3rd year
3 months orthopaedics
9 months basic science

4th year
6 months adult orthopaedics
6 months pediatric orthopaedics

5th year (senior resident)
6 months adult orthopaedics
6 months pediatric orthopaedics

Akron's lack of academic accouterments, satisfying the basic science requirement by obtaining two slots at the University of Pennsylvania's Graduate School of Medicine through the cooperation of Jesse T. Nicholson, professor of orthopaedics at Penn. City Hospital paid the $1,500 tuition, but not living expenses. Residents supported themselves by working in the emergency rooms or as night residents on call. Interest free loans were available, supported by funding from Akron City's medical staff.

James W. Parks, City, class of '49, was the first to attend Penn. Another early graduate, Walter H. Brown, M.D., City, class of '48, graduated from the University of Louisville's School of Medicine in 1940 and was a junior attending on City Hospital's staff in 1946. Both Parks and Brown were Board Certified in orthopaedics and were members of the American Academy of Orthopaedic Surgeons, the Ohio Orthopaedic Society, and the American College of Surgeons. Brown practiced for many years with George Bischoff

The medical profession was a small world then. Hoyt's choice of residency came about through a meeting with Duke's director of the Department of Orthopaedics, Lenox Baker. The Drs. Hoyt met Dr. Baker at a Clinical Orthopaedic Society conference in 1946 and the senior Hoyt introduced his son: "Where are you?" Baker asked. "I'm nowhere," Hoyt, Jr. replied, "I just got out of the army." "I'll hire you," Baker said. "No CV, nothing," Hoyt recalled years later. "Just I'll hire you, when do you want to start? I went down to Durham a couple months later to begin my residency."

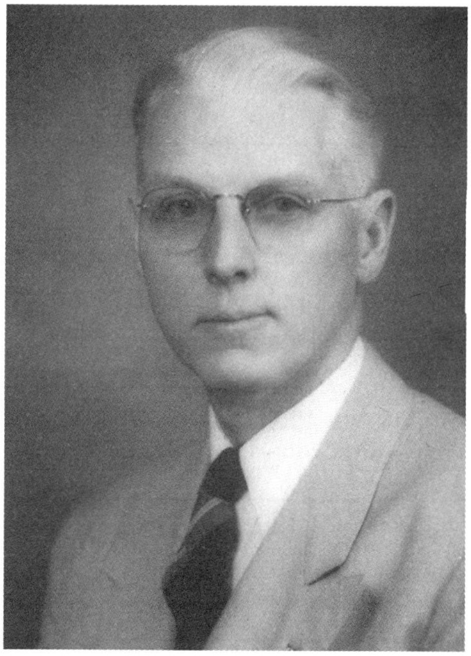

Fowler B. Roberts. Specialists were few and times were tough in the late 1930's when Dr. Roberts returned from the University of Pennsylvania Graduate School of Medicine and confined his practice to orthopaedics.

and Adrian E. Davis and Parks practiced with William M. Davis.

The year at the University of Pennsylvania's Graduate School of Medicine exposed residents to some talented orthopaedists. Jesse T. Nicholson once hosted a dinner for the residents and their instructors. Guests included Paul Colonna, famed for his arthroplasty of the hip, John Royal Moore of Temple University, an advocate of delayed fracture treatment, Anthony DePalma, author of a book on the shoulder, and Al Shands of the DuPont Institute in Wilmington, Delaware.

Residents attended Nicholson's OR and clinic sessions at Penn and the Children's Hospital of Philadelphia. Moore's Tuesday morning fracture clinics were a "must," as were his surgical sessions at the Shriners Hospital. Another "must" on the rotation: DePalma's orthopaedic conferences in the "Pit" at Jefferson - followed by lunch at Bookbinders, oysters on the half shell, ship's biscuit, and a beer. One semester, the residents attended Dr. Shands' Thursday afternoon conferences at the A.I. Dupont Institute in Wilmington, Delaware. Shands treated a broad variety of pediatric orthopaedic patients and brought many of them to these conferences.

Resident training was, and is, rigorous and exhausting. Senior residents provided major care on the wards and participated in surgery subject to the approval and assistance of the attending physician. Senior residents also prepared to take Part One of the certifying board examination, a two day ordeal consisting of written and oral examinations developed and administered by the American Board of Orthopaedic Surgery. Satisfactory completion of this examination was a requirement for appointment to the staff of most teaching hospitals.

George J. Mallo, M.D., City, class of '63 recalls the University of Pennsylvania basic science sojourn. "The hospital did not pay our salaries in Pennsylvania, but they did provide interest-free loans. That's different from what it is today. Now they get paid for everything." Residents received about $150 per month in the forties. Annual compensation for house staff starts at $32,000 in 1997.

As senior resident performing a mid-dorsal spinal fusion on a patient of W.A. Hoyt, Jr., Bill Davis had a scare and learned a lesson. As one lamina was being prepared to receive a bone graft, the small gouge penetrated the lamina causing a major extension reflex. Badly shaken, Davis tried to give the instruments back to the attending, who refused them. "You started the case," Hoyt said, "you finish it." Davis did so, after a look under the lamina revealed only a small laceration in the covering dura. He spent the rest of the day in the patient's room (no recovery room then), leaving only when he was reassured that all reflexes and muscle activity in the lower extremities were normal.

The hospital paid interns $30 per month in those days and provided their "whites," and room and board. The intern's responsibilities included morning blood rounds and IV medications. Interns and residents were on call every other night. The hospitals did not have around-the-clock laboratory technicians until the late forties, so house officers did routine lab work after 5:00 pm. Nighttime X-rays waited until the on-call X-ray technician was summoned from home and drove to the hospital. House staff took and developed the film themselves when there was great urgency.

Bill Davis recalls a $15 bonus "if your charts were all complete. It was an onerous job," he continued, "with the patient gone home, to sit down and write a summary of the case on a chart, particularly if you hadn't been to bed in three days. When the Gray House (house staff's quarters) was demolished, they found incomplete files up in the corners of the attic, files that had been missing probably since my days as a resident."

Polio

Throughout the 1940's and into the 1950's, infantile paralysis continued to cast a pall over summer. It was a major concern of orthopaedists and, hence, a major part of residency training. Retired spine surgeon, Daniel Bethem, City, class of '77, says that "there is no disease that has had as great an impact on orthopaedic surgery. Polio treatment required the accurate assessment of muscle and joints and fastidious attention to repeated evaluations along with maintaining joint motion and ambulation..." Bethem concluded by recognizing "those Akron surgeons who spent long hours tending to these polio patients... They included Walter Hoyt, Sr., Fowler Roberts, Edwin Mollin, Walter Hoyt, Jr., Donald Minnig, and Harry O'Dell."

Children's Hospital was designated as one of several Polio Centers for the State of Ohio in 1944 and admitted roughly 20 percent of all polio patients in the state. Treatment for the most part was conservative, bracing and physical therapy being the first lines of defense. Approximately 10 to 15 percent of patients required reconstructive surgery to relieve contractions and deformities which had developed due to muscle imbalance and weakness.

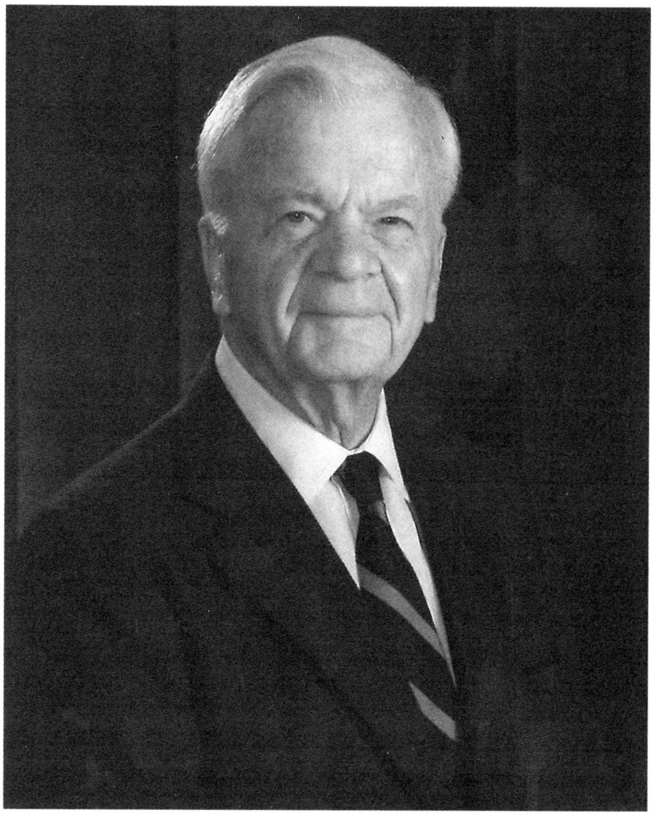

Walter A. Hoyt, Jr. Dr. Hoyt encouraged many talented young clinicians to practice in Akron and they helped build the solid foundation of education and research that is essential to high quality patient care. **Summa Health System**

The Goodyear blimp rumbled overhead in the summer and fall of 1947, its illuminated signs flashing the polio admissions count in the worst epidemic yet, 415 patients admitted to Children's. So many, that neighboring Grace Evangelical and Reformed Church took the overflow patients in their basement, which had been converted into a hospital ward. Grace Evangelical Church opened again in 1952 when in-house polio patients totaled over six hundred.

W.A. Hoyt Jr.'s 1949 arrival in Akron coincided with a polio epidemic. Akron's orthopaedists often bring back new procedures. New techniques in the surgical management of polio was Hoyt's first "bring back." In a 1997 interview, he told of his good fortune to have trained at Duke where he had the opportunity to work under the surgeons at Warm Springs, Georgia [a research and treatment facility specializing in polio]. There he learned a tremendous amount about the surgical management of patients with poliomyelitis and shared this Warm Springs experience with the residents and staff in Akron.

In that same interview, he recalled going to Children's after a full day in the office and the operating room during the 1949 through 1952 polio epidemics. "I'd start out around seven in the evening with a couple residents and a nurse, make rounds, examine patients, and recommend continuing treatment, including physical therapy and use of braces. Surgical management of polio was undertaken after the patient had had extensive physical therapy and bracing. When patients reached a point where they couldn't make any more progress and where we felt that we could get rid of their braces and improve their functional capability, then we would do surgery. We'd do tendon transplants, fusions, growth arrests, and other bony and soft tissue operations to strengthen their extremities and improve their functional capacity."

A bit of fun boosts morale. *Life* magazine carried a small article in 1952 featuring Children's Hospital's colorful plaster casts. Charles Houck, M.D., City, class of '52, liberated a supply of Easter egg coloring dye from the hospital's kitchen and dyed the water in which he dipped plaster for casts. Children's blossomed, Dr. Bill Davis recalls, in "assorted colors of spicas, club foot, and fracture casts. Some were in two or more hues."

A.E. Davis succeeds W.A. Hoyt, Sr. at City

Adrian E. Davis was chosen director of City's orthopaedic surgery division in 1949 following Walter A. Hoyt Sr's. death. A fellow of the American College of Surgeons, Davis was a bootstrap orthopaedist (no residency in orthopaedics), as were Hoyt, Sr. and F. B. Roberts. A.E. Davis's tenure ran through the fifties, when, as Zouhair Yassine says, "plaster of Paris was the orthopaedist's best friend and was not relegated to the orthopaedic technician." Residents continued to receive their basic science courses at the University of Pennsylvania Graduate School of Medicine.

Davis concentrated on education, with City's junior and senior attendings comprising the teaching staff. Junior staff had completed their residencies and were required to complete two years of practice before taking the second part of the Board examinations. The junior staff's duties included attending the charity clinics in rotation and assisting and teaching the residents. If a patient was scheduled for surgery out of that clinic, the attending staff physician was required to be present during the procedure, a practice that still prevails.

The Monday Noon Conference, held in the eighth floor solarium of what is now Surgical East, was the only "classroom" activity from the program's outset through the fifties and early sixties. Residents chose and presented cases and demonstrated new procedures for staff critique. The attendings whose cases were up for discussion were notified and the prudent attending made sure he was on hand to defend his clinical management. Errors and complications were on the agenda, too, making the conference an

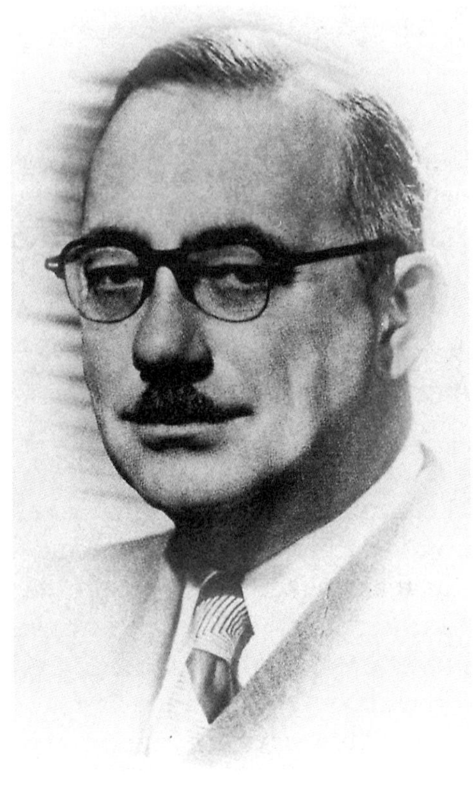

Adrian E. Davis. Dr. Davis was in his first year as Director of City's orthopaedic residency program when he was tapped to be the hospital's Chief of Staff in 1950.

excellent tool for peer review and quality control.

Visiting professors are a valuable educational resource. In the early sixties, the orthopaedic staff combined television, a marvelous instructional medium, with a visiting professor. They invited Bill Stewart, a disciple of Paul Harrington's, to come to Children's Hospital and perform a scoliosis fusion with Harrington instrumentation on closed-circuit television. Harrington had published his work utilizing spinal instrumentation in 1960, but acceptance was slow, according to Daniel Bethem. Roger Burke, owner of radio and television station WAKR, arranged the close-circuit televising of the surgery, which was broadcast to Children's auditorium.

A host of medical personnel and the Children's Hospital Women's Board witnessed Akron's first closed-circuit televised surgery. "The only aspect of the event that created a problem," according to Bethem, "was Dr. Stewart's very colorful language." As W.A. Hoyt would recall years later, "Bill Stewart didn't know how to talk without swearing." "Stewart's frequent expletives created some consternation among the Women's Board members," said Bethem, who concludes, "Harrington instrumentation made an auspicious entry into the armamentarium of the orthopaedic service in Akron, Ohio."

A New Residency in Orthopaedic Surgery

Akron's second orthopaedic's residency program was set up at General (formerly Peoples) Hospital in the 1950's by the four senior attending orthopaedic surgeons of that institution, Donald I. Minnig, Edwin Mollin, Harry O'Dell, and Fowler B. Roberts. The American Board of Orthopaedic Surgery's Residency Review Committee certified the program in 1957. The ABOS required one year of training in general surgery, one year of adult orthopaedics, one year pediatric orthopaedics, six months of fractures and six months of basic science.

Scientific medicine had been in its toddling stage when Peoples Hospital opened on West Cedar Street in 1915. Laboratories were just then becoming essential to a well equipped hospital and Peoples lab was duly listed after the number of beds and staff in newspaper accounts. A more interesting feature, according to the *Akron Beacon Journal*, was "three porches with southern exposure, each enclosed in glass which can be removed at will." Fresh air, sunlight, nourishing food, not technology or research, held sway in those days.

Things had changed forty years later; research was a hot topic. People's changed its name in 1955 to Akron General Hospital - and its address - when a major building program added 177 beds and moved the hospital's main entrance from Cedar Street to Wabash Avenue. The new building contained a research laboratory and in 1960, Harry W. O'Dell became General's first director of research. Though an improvement over that first tiny lab, facilities were limited, according to Buel S. Smith, M.D. Nevertheless, O'Dell showed that worthwhile research could be done in a community hospital, as he developed the first bone research laboratory in this area. Later, according to Dr. O'Dell, General's laboratory would feature "pioneer work in the treatment of shock by Dr. James Berk."

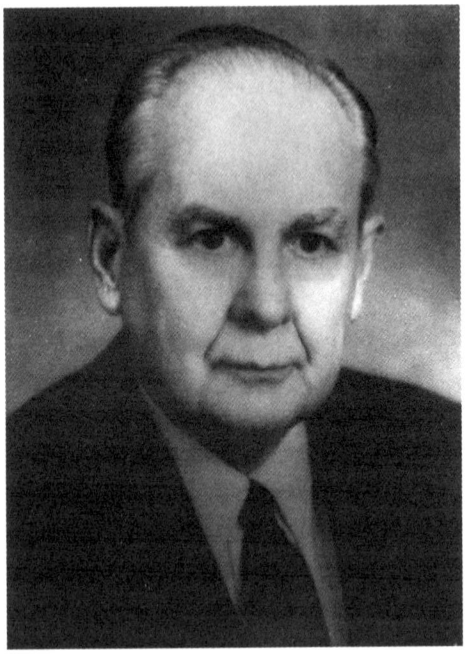

Harry O'Dell. Dr. O'Dell, chairman of Akron General's Department of Orthopaedics from 1963 to 1974, played a vital role in the development of education and research in Akron General Medical Center's residency in orthopaedic surgery. **Akron General Medical Center**

Having dealt with bricks and mortar, Akron General Hospital's Board of Trustees, chaired by Frank Steere, turned to strengthening the hospital as an educational institution. Chairman Steere appointed a long range planning committee chaired by Dr. O'Dell, with Trustees Al Howland and Willard Bear, Dr. Robert Allison from Administration, and Dr. Henry Kraus from the staff as members. According to Buel Smith, "Dr. O'Dell has always had an aversion to committees of all types, but especially to large committees." O'Dell reviewed General's educational program and recommended that a committee of five, composed of two trustees, two physicians, and the President of Akron General Hospital, have total control of the training programs, such as the new residency in orthopaedic surgery. According to Dr. Smith, this Trustees Committee on Medical Education represented "a radical change in the hospital's power structure, but was eventually accepted by the medical staff and the trustees."

Medicine did not escape change in the fractious sixties, a time of upheavals, protests, and generational clashes. The federal government attacked the medical establishment, calling it a "cottage industry," which turned out far fewer doctors than the country needed. Locally, problems with intern recruitment in the fifties and sixties threatened Akron General's growing educational program, according to Buel Smith. Harry O'Dell was appointed intern recruitment director in 1959 and successfully recruited the hospital's quota of twenty. Three of that class became orthopaedic surgeons, including Alan Holderness, who was interim chief of orthopaedics in 1974.

The success of 1959 did not solve the problem of a shortage of qualified students, however, and both of Akron's orthopaedic residency programs experienced recruiting difficulties into the sixties. Medical students were in short supply and the siren song of the glamour specialty, general surgery, often lured away prospects. Akron's Children's Hospital, nationally known and highly regarded, was recruiting's one bright spot. Buel Smith recalls that Children's drew medical students to the Rubber City at a time when "competition for residents was intense among the orthopaedic residencies, and it is reasonably certain that, in time, Akron's orthopaedic surgery residencies would have disappeared, except for one fact. That fact was the decision made in the late 1920's that all pediatric patients would be concentrated in a separate institution, namely Children's Hospital. Many students sought residency training in Akron primarily because our programs were strong in pediatric orthopaedics."

Two residents were accepted into General's program each year, as at City's. Now that Akron's community hospitals offered two orthopaedic residencies, there was a shortage of places for all the residents in pediatric orthopaedics at Children's. For a time, one General resident went to Children's, the other to Gates Memorial Children's Hospital in Elyria, Ohio, where Dr. Clarence Heymon, an internationally known orthopaedist, was the surgeon-in-chief. Later, both went to Akron Children's. Both programs' residents took the academic "year at Penn" until 1964 when the program directors decided to teach basic science locally.

The physician influencing many of these changes at Akron General, Harry W. O'Dell, has had a distinguished career as a clinician, teacher, and researcher. Dr. O'Dell received his A.B. at Indiana University in 1942, his M.D. at Indiana University in 1944, and a M.Msc at the University of Pennsylvania in 1952. He took residencies at the Medical Center in New Jersey, University of Pennsylvania, and the Cleveland Clinic. He was chief of orthopaedic surgery at Camp Lee Regional Hospital during the Second World War.

Dr. O'Dell first chaired the orthopaedic service in 1954 when it was a general surgery division. Even today, in some institutions, orthopaedics is a service of general surgery, not a department. According to Dr. Smith, "despite considerable opposition, Dr. O'Dell won the necessary support to change this status to a separate department. His efforts greatly increased the influence of orthopaedic surgery within the hospital." What had been a division was now a major service, along with general surgery, medicine, and obstetrics. Without this important change in status, Smith concludes, "it is difficult to believe that the department would have developed as it has."

The department's first chairman, Donald I. Minnig, served from 1957 to 1960. He was succeeded by Fowler B. Roberts, who served from 1960 to 1962. Dr. Roberts retired in the mid-sixties after a distinguished career in orthopaedic surgery. His son, James D. Roberts, M.D., recalls that his father's

Following his chairmanship of the department, Dr. Roberts established the F.B. Roberts Lecture in orthopaedic surgery, which continues on an annual basis. Dr. O'Dell selected and sponsored the speakers, the first being Dr. David Dahlin of the Mayo Clinic in 1967. The Second Annual F.B. Roberts Lecture on May 8, 1968, was by Dr. Robert P. Heaney, Professor of Medicine, Creighton University School of Medicine. Leonard F. Peltier, M.D., of the University of Kansas Medical Center delivered the third lecture on November 5, 1969, and Rocco A. Calandruccio, M.D., of the Campbell Clinic in Memphis, Tennessee, delivered the fourth annual lecture.

modification of a surgical technique was published in the July 1944 issue of the *Journal of the Ohio State Medical Association.*

Over the years, Akron physicians forged bonds through the city's two orthopaedic residencies. Consider for a moment who founded these programs. Children's chief of staff, W.S. Chase served on Peoples' building committee and brought W.A. Hoyt, Sr. to Akron in 1916 to organize Children's Department of Orthopaedic Surgery. Fowler B. Roberts, a founder of General's orthopaedic residency, took an orthopaedic preceptorship with Hoyt, Sr. in 1928 and worked with him in 1946 to establish City/Children's combined residency. Today, Mark Leeson and Patrick Flanagan, General's and Summa's department chairmen respectively, co-operate on a host of matters affecting the residencies.

Building an Educational Infrastructure in Akron

American orthopaedics, Akron orthopaedics, and the local residency programs experienced many changes in the twenty years during which Walter Asahel Hoyt, Jr. directed the specialty at City and Children's Hospitals. Few high quality text books were available in the sixties and only two orthopaedic journals were peer reviewed. The area lacked a medical school for the first half of Hoyt's tenure, as well as a laboratory devoted to musculoskeletal research. Dennis Weiner recalls that research projects were "funded out of pocket (the doctor's pocket)."

Akron's orthopaedists began strengthening the local educational infrastructure in 1964 when, instead of sending residents to the University of Pennsylvania's Graduate School of Medicine, Hoyt and O'Dell brought them home for basic science. Both men believed, according to Harry O'Dell, "that basic science training in Akron would not only benefit the residents, but also the staff and community." The "year at Penn" was over.

Dr. O'Dell directed the basic science program. Over the years, Sam Barley, Whit Ewing, and Dennis Weiner taught pathology. Zouhair Yassine was chief instructor of anatomy and also taught the Swiss method of ORIF. First held on Thursday evenings, this combined basic science program later

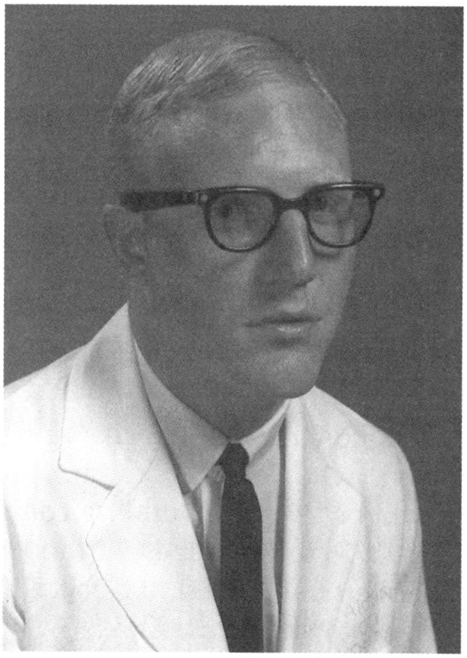

E. Herbert Thompson, photographed here as an intern at City, has served as a team physician at the University of Akron for many years. **Summa Health System**

moved to Saturday mornings at Children's under the direction of Dennis Weiner. Dr. Hoyt recalled other orthopaedic surgeons who taught basic science: George Mallo, Buel Smith, Herbert Thompson, Barry Greenberg, and J. Patrick Flanagan.

At the turn of the century, Charles B. Nancrede (Hoyt, Sr.'s teacher) had recruited promising medical school students as his assistants; they were on his service and lived at the University of Michigan's hospital during their senior year. Akron's orthopaedists followed a similar plan in building their programs. As W.A. Hoyt, Jr. said in an interview in 1997, "we needed young people with exceptional talent to join us, help with the teaching, help with the research, and build up the department as a whole. We had to develop teachers. We didn't have all these well educated subspecialists [in the sixties]. We had to educate them, or get them educated, so they could come back and be part of the active teaching staff. We wanted experts who were full time in pediatric orthopaedics, expert hand surgeons, a hand service. And not only did we want experts in all the subspecialties, we wanted them to have adequate space for research and teaching. Now, the people who took specialty training after their residency are around here today [1997] and have a leading role in these hospital-based residency programs and in our medical school."

These goals took years to achieve. Ivan A. Gradisar, Jr., City, class of '72,

Flanagan, who grew up in Columbus, Ohio, chose City for his residency during the hospital's 1966 September Day program for senior medical students. "A fellow classmate from Akron suggested I attend; City had the reputation of being one of the two best community hospitals in Ohio." His September Day group included a medical student from the University of Iowa, one from the University of Cincinnati, and one from the University of West Virginia. Ewing, recently returned from Vietnam after a tour as general medical officer for the U.S. Marines, guided the quartet around the hospital. "Dr. Ewing sported a Drill Instructor haircut and had a persona to match," Flanagan later remembered. He supposed this commanding individual was City's chief surgical resident. Not so, said Dr. Robert Bartlett, then chairman of the Department of General Surgery. "Dr. Ewing was a first year orthopaedic resident rotating on general surgery who acted as if he was chief resident of the hospital."

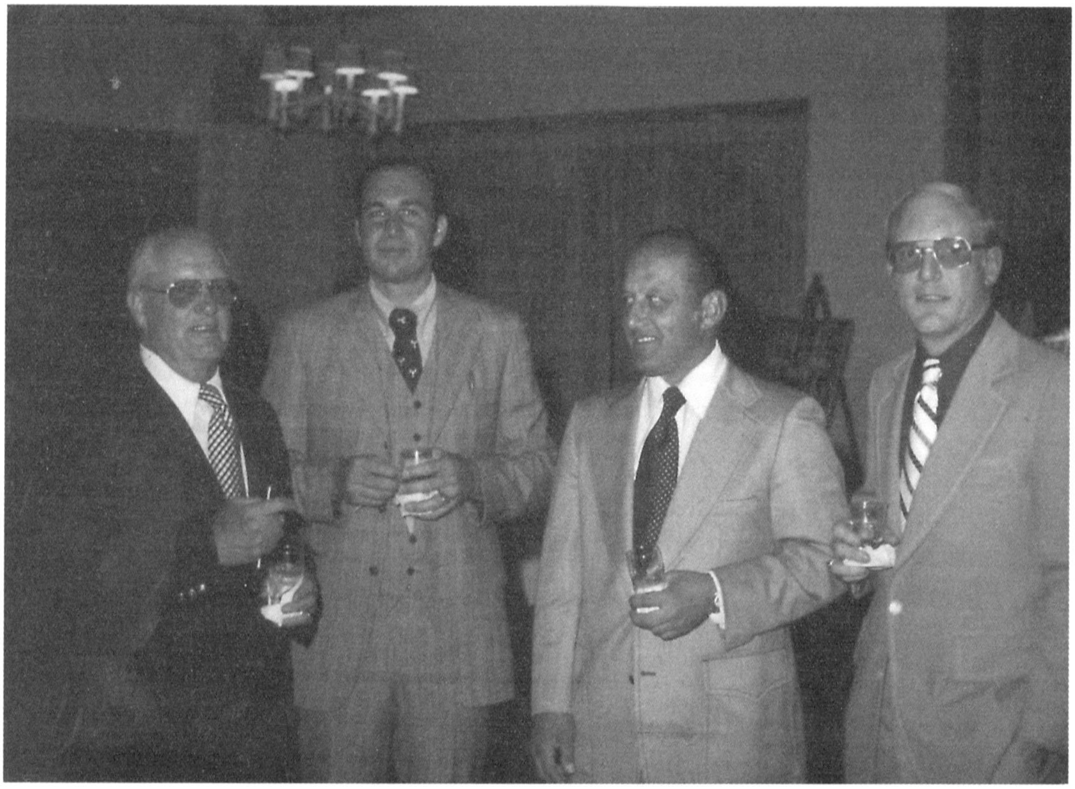

Left to Right, Drs. Walter Brown, Henry Hood, George Mallo, and Herbert Thompson at a Hoyt Society resident conference in 1981. Dr. Hood collects old orthopaedic text books and instruments and travels the globe distributing them to physicians in the third world.
Summa Health System

and J. Patrick Flanagan, City, class of '73 are two whose experience shows how the residencies have grown since the sixties. Then, "education was primarily on-the-job training," Dr. Flanagan recalls. "When I arrived in 1968, there was one weekly fracture conference, a 'show and tell.'" (Which, according to Dr. Hoyt, was popular with the residents and orthopaedic staff - "they'd get up and scream at each other.") "Dr. Henry Hood was Chief Resident," Flanagan said. "He quickly became a role model, as did Dr. Whit Ewing. Dr. Ewing had an extreme gift of intuitive diagnostic capabilities and he certainly fit the image of the orthopaedist in personality, including his nickname 'Iron Hands.'"

Ivan Gradisar was in the last group of orthopaedic residents to intern in general surgery. He recalls that he, Roger Lane, and Frank Forshew "rotated through all the conventional surgical services, including running the emergency room for twenty-four hours on, twenty-four hours off. Sometimes you had the help of an orthopaedic resident, or some other resident, if you had a difficult case. It was a beast of a call; you were almost guaranteed to be sick when the month's rotation was over. In October, 1967, in twenty-four hours, we saw one hundred patients in City's ER. It's my understanding that they

Gradisar also recalls that, given his strong committment to research and education, Hoyt "was a tyrant with any resident who speculated about the interesting academic options of care at the patient's bedside. He insisted that the patient be treated with dignity and respect and be presented with a clear and well conceived treatment plan carried out with attention to the most minute detail." The Chairman often gave very pointed lessons in good grooming, another way of showing respect for patients. Gradisar recalls that "the resident who showed up on the wards without a clean white shirt, uniform, and tie and clean shaven, was also in trouble. One Saturday morning in 1968 while making rounds he caught me eyeing his blue dress shirt. He looked over and said, 'it's the only blue one I own.'"

still see 120 patients in twenty-four hours, but now they have full-time emergency room physicians, residents, and staff who do the same work."

Despite the lack of laboratory facilities, Akron's orthopaedic residents did research in the 1960's. Flanagan and Gradisar conducted animal experiments in which they demonstrated the mechanism of air embolism from subclavian venipuncture. Dr. Flanagan received the Walter A. Hoyt Award for Basic Science Research for this work. The award, honoring the senior Hoyt, was established in 1958 to encourage and reward residents for basic research in all medical fields. While a resident, Dr. Flanagan also did some original work on injecting cortisone into tendons.

In addition to maintaining a busy practice in Akron, Dr. Hoyt's national experience and outlook has had a strong, positive influence on City's orthopaedic residency program. He served his specialty nationally through the American Academy of Orthopaedic Surgeons. His AAOS career began in the late fifties as a member of the Regional Committee (now the Board of Counselors) and culminated in 1973-74 as President of the Academy. Over the years, he recalls having served "on every single board, every single organization nationally that had any thing to do with orthopaedic education." As Dr. Gradisar once said, "Dr. Hoyt has never taken his eye off the academic ball."

Three Essential Elements: The E.M.T., The M.D., The R.N.

Medical Doctors constitute one part of the health care team. Emergency Medical Technicians transport the maimed and the sick to the hospital and, once there, Registered Nurses provide care. Medical knowledge has grown so rapidly over the last half century, that these three essential elements have undergone great change in learning to take care of patients. We begin with the doctors.

Continuing medical education is a given today. Certification and recertification are part of medical practice. This was not the case in the early sixties when Walter A. Hoyt, Jr. joined the AAOS's new Committee on Injuries, chaired by Dr. Sam Banks. The committee's goal: improve orthopaedic surgeons' knowledge in the field of trauma. "We sent out flyers," Hoyt recalled, "asking them to come, spend three days listening to lectures on all the current knowledge and techniques in relation to trauma." Formal continuing medical education in orthopaedics began in 1964 at that first postgraduate course for orthopaedists, held in Atlanta, Georgia, under the direction of Dr. Wood Lovell. Eventually, the Committee on Injuries had thirty-six courses in all phases of orthopaedics going on around the country.

Not all doctors enthusiastically embraced certification in the sixties; some were downright antagonistic to recertification. A comprehensive Academy study, "*National Health Program for Orthopaedics*," was quashed in 1969 because one sentence in the appendix suggested that accountability and recertification of orthopaedists might be considered in the future. "I've never seen such a hew and cry," Hoyt recalled. "They just picked that (sentence) up and they just tore it out. The committee had to withdraw (the report) and make an official apology." Stung by the rejection, the American Board of Orthopaedic Surgery waited a decade before conducting a "trial" recertification examination.

Emergency Medicine

Procedures once considered impossible became technically feasible in the 1960's and, on June 22, 1964, six Akron surgeons, led by Harry O'Dell, performed one of the area's first, if not the first, replantation. An eight-year-old boy was brought from Lodi Hospital to Children's Hospital following complete severance of the midshaft of the lower leg by a mowing machine. The amputated limb was recovered in the field by the family's doctor and arrived at Children's in a bucket of ice. The surgical team worked five hours replanting the leg, which was viable for several days. Unfortunately, the veins thrombosed and the lower portion was lost.

Akronites considered this replantation case a miracle. Given the state of emergency services at the time, the patient's arrival at Children's was a wonder in itself. The farm had no phone, so the family could not call an ambulance, which, in those days, was a "low, flat car in which it was impossible to stand, or even kneel," Dr. Hoyt said. "Therefore, it was impossible to administer life support on the way to the hospital. They could occasionally give oxygen, but even that was difficult." There were no interstate highways. Rescuers ran to the local road, flagged down a car, drove six miles to the Lodi Hospital where physicians stabilized the boy and he was taken to Children's. Today, a call to 911 would have trained personnel on the scene in minutes and the patient would be life-flighted to Children's.

In 1964, the AAOS's Committee on Injuries, then chaired by Walter

Hoyt, developed a program to train emergency medical technicians. Entitled "emergency care and transportation of the sick and injured," the course contained a huge amount of information to impart to non-physicians, some of whom had only a high school education. They needed a text book, "with a lot of illustrations and an educational program where students could take a six month's course, have a regular curriculum," Hoyt said. "That's what's happened throughout the country now." Zouhair Yassine ran the first two courses for paramedics offered at the University of Akron. Another change: those low, flat ambulances assumed the boxy configuration so familiar today.

Emergency Care and Transportation of the Sick and Injured, first published in 1971 by the American Academy of Orthopaedic Surgeons, under Dr. Hoyt's supervision, has strong connections with Akron's orthopaedic residency programs. Dennis Weiner recalls that "orthopaedic residents from General and City worked with the Bath (Ohio) Township Fire and Rescue Squad developing this emergency medicine manual." Led by Chief Larry Hershey, Bath's fire fighters helped construct the courses for the manual. "They were wonderful," Dr. Weiner said of Bath's prototype E.M.T. personnel, "they helped give the courses and worked with the emergency medical people." Bath Township rescue squad members are pictured in *Emergency Care,* demonstrating "regular lifts and carries," "special lifts and carries," and "types of stretchers and their uses."

Many knowledgeable people contributed to writing *Emergency Care,* which was an immediate success. It has gone through several revisions, sold over five million copies, and generated more than $20 million for the Academy. A Massachusetts police officer, John B. Palmer, a veteran of what he terms "the old snatch and grab days" of ambulance work, appreciated the manual "because they didn't talk down to us, but they didn't talk as though we were a bunch of doctors, either."

The Nurses

Robert J. White, M.D., Professor of Neurosurgery at Case Western Reserve University's School of Medicine, Director of Neurological Surgery and of the Brain Research Laboratory at Cleveland's MetroHealth Medical Center, says that "Doctors diagnose and operate; doctors prescribe drugs. But the hour-to-hour vigilance and care of the sick is the true responsibility of the nurse." Writing about the nursing profession in the *Beacon Journal*'s Guest Viewpoint column, April 9, 1996, Dr. White said that "without nurses in our major medical health facilities, regardless of the level of biotechnological sophistication, few severely injured or ill patients would survive. Far more than the physician's involvement, the one-on-one care provided by the nurse to the sickest, the elderly, and the poor is the basic reason a patient will be

Dr. Bill Davis recalls hearing medical futurist, Leland Keiser, Ph.D., puzzle and astound his physician audience by asking why patients entered the hospital. "After getting varied answers, Dr. Keiser told us, 'patients enter the hospital because they need NURSING CARE. Most illnesses are cared for in the home - most surgery is out-patient. Only when nursing care is needed does the patient come into the hospital.' Keiser then suggested we all go back to our hospitals and say 'thank you' to the nurses caring for our patients."

cured or his or her quality of life extended."

Nurses are essential to quality patient care and they also do a good deal of informal teaching, "often first under the gun in educating our residents," according to Davis. One reviewer of City's orthopaedic residency program's early days noted approvingly on his report that "not one traction bed was in disarray." The nursing staff would have it no other way.

Nurses rose in those days whenever a doctor entered the station; each wore her "cap," proudly recognizing her school of nursing. Times change. Medical procedures change. Jean Morton, R.N. recalls the days of "turpentine stupes and molasses enemas...the old oxygen tanks that had to be filled with ice and monitored almost as closely as the patient." But, some things do not change, Mrs. Morton says, "not the basic principles of good total patient care. Things you learn as a probationer that stay with you always;" for one, "the close relationship you develop with the patient and the patient's family."

A graduate of Good Samaritan Hospital's School of Nursing in Sandusky, Mrs. Morton came to City Hospital for a refresher course in 1965 after a long absence from the field. She completed the course, applied for a nursing position, and requested a medical floor. A family member had been diagnosed with diabetes "and I wanted to learn anything new in diabetes." There were no openings on a medical floor, so she went to orthopaedics, and took to it so enthusiastically that she retired as head nurse of Three East in 1978 with honorary membership in the Department of Orthopaedics.

Told she would have two weeks orientation in orthopaedics, an area new to her, Mrs. Morton was assigned to Hazel Conlon's floor, Three West, a forty-two bed unit. Help was short on Three West and Mrs. Conlon recognized

A lot of traction was used in the sixties and, "if you're new to orthopaedics," Mrs. Morton said, "it's rough to learn. Every traction is different." Mrs. Conlon held classes on the various tractions: Right and Left Balanced Suspension with Pearson Attachments, Russell's Traction, Pelvic Traction, Head Halters, and how to handle cervical fractures and dislocations. "What a frightening experience, the first time I cared for a patient with Skull Tongs inserted."

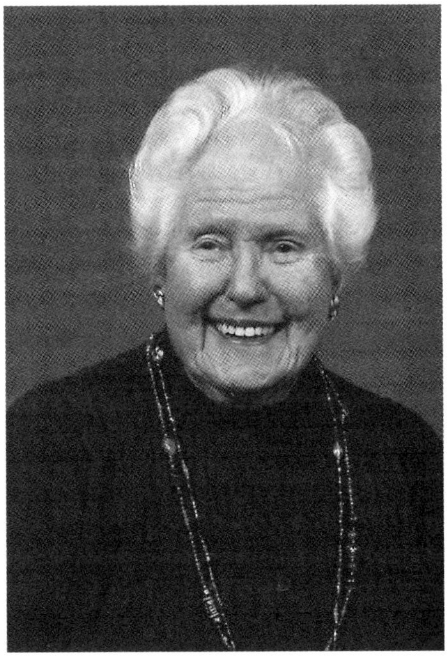

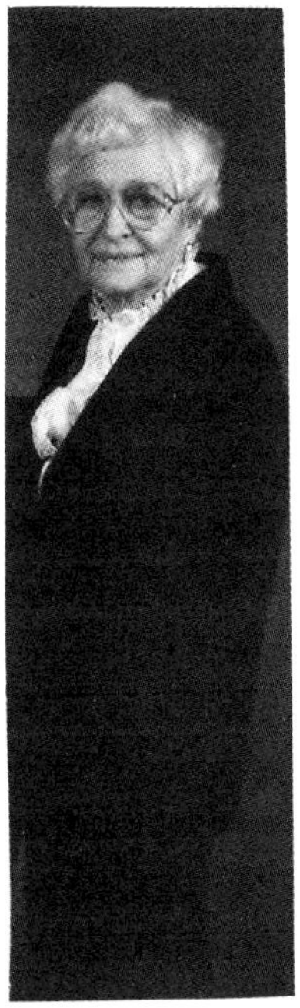

Hazel Conlon, R.N. and Jean Morton, R.N. Mrs. Conlon and Mrs. Morton experienced and adapted to a host of technological changes in their nursing careers. But, as Mrs. Morton has observed, one thing remained constant: "the basic principles of good total patient care."

Photos supplied by Mrs. Conlon and Mrs. Morton

leadership ability when she saw it. Though Mrs. Morton had been on the ward only two days, Mrs. Conlon knew she could take a team, that is, lead a group of nurses in caring for patients. And, despite initial misgivings on Morton's part, she did. (As an orthopaedics nurse, she also "soon learned that diabetes was a big factor in many patients' care.")

Mrs. Morton became Mrs. Conlon's assistant, then followed Dorothy Bennett, R.N. as head nurse on thirty-six bed Three East. Mary A. Evancho was her assistant. Mrs. Evancho became Head Nurse of Three West when Mrs. Conlon retired in 1972. Summa Health System's Orthopaedic Nursing Unit, now at St. Thomas Hospital, is dedicated to Mrs. Evancho's memory. Speaking at the dedication, Patrick Flanagan, chairman of the Department of Orthopaedic Surgery, said of Mrs. Evancho, "she practiced nursing with unselfish dedication to the service of others and was most definitely a leader. Compassion for the sick and suffering was her only motive as she fought for her patients and for her nursing staff with boundless energy."

The head nurse's job, according to Mrs. Morton, is "a twenty-four-hour a day concern. We work different shifts to see how people are functioning. You soon know who's dependable, who's giving good care - and who's goofing off."

Every job has its downsides. Mrs. Morton's list includes "the never ending, never relenting fight against decubiti [pressure sores]; the hunt when patients left dentures, eye glasses, even coin purses on diet trays; getting each shift to clean their isolation rooms before the next shift took over; absenteeism and tardiness; unacceptable conditions discovered on surprise bed pan and sterilizer inspections." Of this last, the head nurse "said to some of the people, would you sit on that pan? I can remember that day. Little things, you know?"

"Hour-to-hour vigilance" is part of nursing's armamentarium and "little things," such as dating the tape when an IV went in service are important. "After morning conference, the nurse on nights and myself went to each patient with an IV," Mrs Morton said, "checked to see if the needle was all right, if it had infiltrated. Dating the tape doesn't seem like much, but it was a lot in patient care."

Another "little thing" in Mrs. Morton's day was "bringing the physical therapist to the units, working with the patients before they were able to be out of bed and go to physical therapy. That was a big advance. Of course, it doesn't sound like much when you think of all the technical advances, but consider the muscles wasting away, the joints getting stiff. Nurses could, and did, help, but we didn't have time to do all the exercises the patient needed."

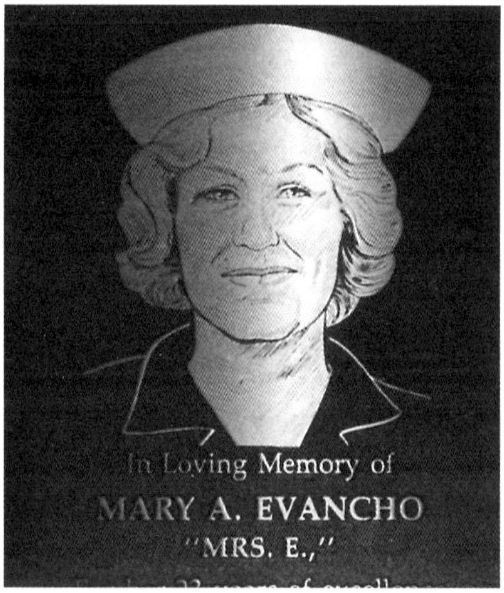

Mary Agnes Evancho, R.N. In today's high-tech medical world, it still is true that "...hour-to-hour vigilance and care of the sick is the true responsibility of the nurse."
Photo by Penny La Bate

How much does a positive attitude count in rehabilitation? According to Mrs. Morton, "90 percent. Some didn't want to do the physical therapy. You found that more in older people. Young people have so many irons in the fire, they're anxious to get going."

Nursing's technical responsibilities have changed and grown tremendously since Mrs. Morton was head nurse of Three East. Nurses do procedures today that only physicians were permitted to do thirty years ago. Mrs. Morton recalled working with Dr. Tom Reef on a patient of Dr. Bill Davis. "This was a Chrysler Plant accident, one of many we treated. The patient had both arms drawn into a roller up to his shoulders. Skin grafting was extensive, the dressings many and bulky. After many days, the patient was making good progress and Dr. Reef decided to go to oral antibiotics. He told me to disconnect the subclavian IV, which I did. Neither of us realized that our instruction manual made no provision for nurses to disconnect subclavian IVs."

Technically, nursing has changed a lot since Bennett, Conlon, Evancho, Morton, and so many others worked their shifts. But, Dr. White's definition of the nurse's "true responsibility" as being "hour to hour vigilance and care of the sick" is just as meaningful today as a century ago. "Successful nursing," Mrs. Morton says, "requires patience, plus caring for the patient. Be concerned, speak encouragement, have compassion, be thoughtful and caring in decision making. Today's nurses are so much more adept and much better educated."

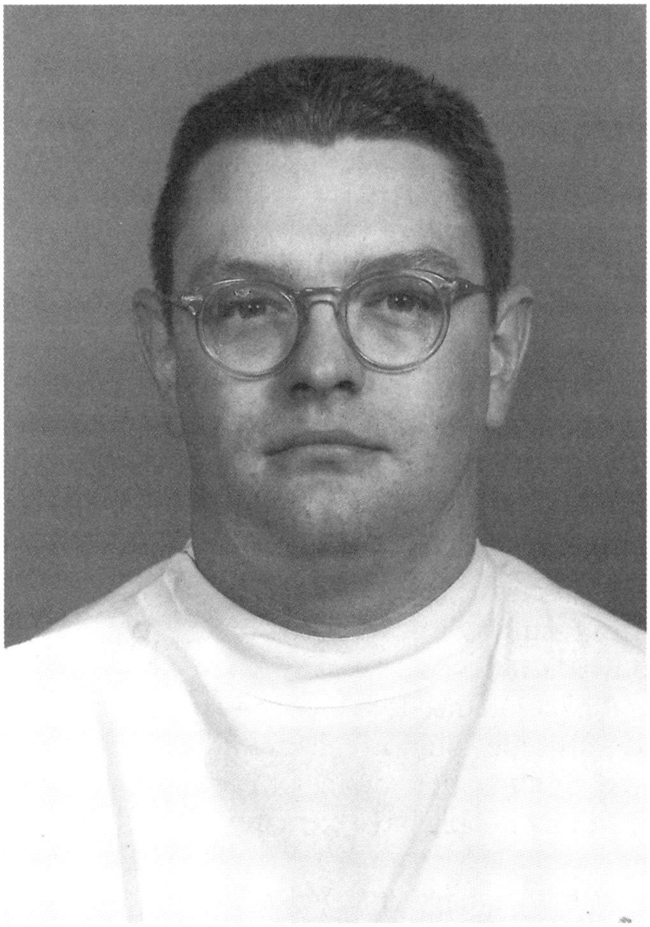

Robert Clark, pictured here as an intern, was a graduate of the University of Michigan Medical School. Dr. Clark served as Head of the Service of City Hospital's Division of Orthopaedic Surgery from 1969 through 1972.
Summa Health System

Asked what advice she would give today's young orthopaedists, Mrs. Morton said, "listen to the patient." She related how she learned to listen to Jimmy, a bright, cerebral palsy patient. "If I looked Jimmy in the eye, I couldn't understand a word he said. But, if I looked past him and let him talk to my ears, I understood every word. Communicate. Let the patient know you care, that you're interested. Let him know that you're interested in his family. They're a big part of the picture and, so many times, they're ignored. Keep on learning. All the avenues of education and research are open to you. These avenues are open to nurses, too. Listen, communicate, keep on learning."

Reorganizing the Programs

As medical knowledge increased in the sixties, residents had more to learn than could be taught trailing the attendings and observing them in the operating room. The residencies required closer attention, tighter control, someone to tend daily operations. The practice of having a part-time chief, elected by his peers, running the department out of his lab coat while maintaining his own practice no longer worked, not if the programs were to keep their accreditation.

Akron General and City reached the same solution — have full-time, hospital-based department chairmen. General's Trustee's Committee on Medical Education, which had total control over its training programs, selected the physicians for these positions. In 1963, City formed its Education Review Committee comprising H. Willard Allison, William Falor, Walter Hoyt, Jr., and C. William Loughrey. In the late sixties, Dr. Andrew J. Kerr (medicine) became City's first full-time hospital-based chairman at this committee's rec-

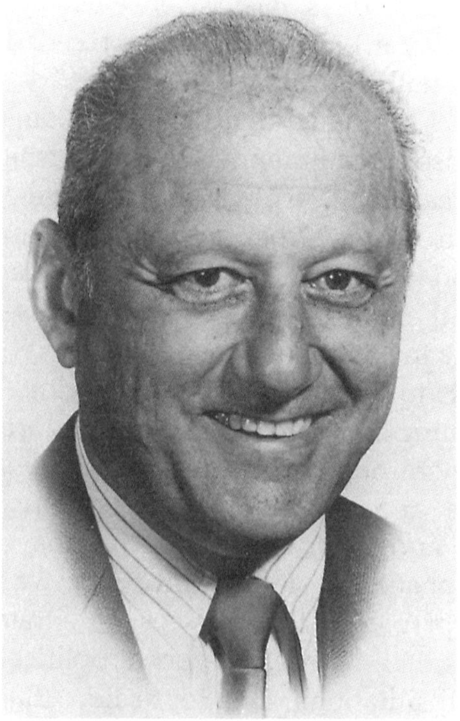

George Mallo, former Chief of Staff at Akron City Hospital in 1979. Now retired, Dr. Mallo recalled his years as a team physician at the University of Akron as being "interesting, fun, and a challenge."
Summa Health System

ommendation.

Dr. Hoyt's AAOS and ABOS duties often took him far away from Akron, reviewing residency programs for the ABOS and monitoring three-day continuing medical education sessions sponsored by the AAOS. He also served on the Board of the National Academy of Sciences and was a consultant to the Department of Transportation and the Department of Health, Education, and Welfare. These national responsibilities expanded exponentially in the sixties. After much discussion, in March, 1969, City's orthopaedic staff unanimously voted to reorganize their division's structure and chain of command. They elected Walter Hoyt Chief of the Division of Orthopaedic Surgery and Robert Clark Head of the Service.

Staff members now became actively involved in administering the residency program. They approved the following committee assignments at their April 29, 1969 meeting:

Committee for Resident Procurement - George Mallo
Committee for Teaching Schedule for the Resident Staff - Buel Smith
Finance Committee - Millard Beyer
Research Committee - William Davis
University of Illinois Project - James Parks
Representatives to Akron General Hospital's Medical Education
Committee - Buel Smith and Robert Clark
Geographical alignment and Resident Education Committee -
Edwin L. Mollin
Resident Interviews - George Mallo

Working together, the orthopaedists fashioned a new educational plan. Dr. Flanagan recalls that "Dr. Buel Smith, then chairman of the Orthopaedic Education Committee at City, established the Saturday morning (fracture) conference schedule which continued for the next twenty-plus years. This conference combined City's and General's orthopaedic residents. That, and basic science, also a combined program given at Children's, comprised formal edu-

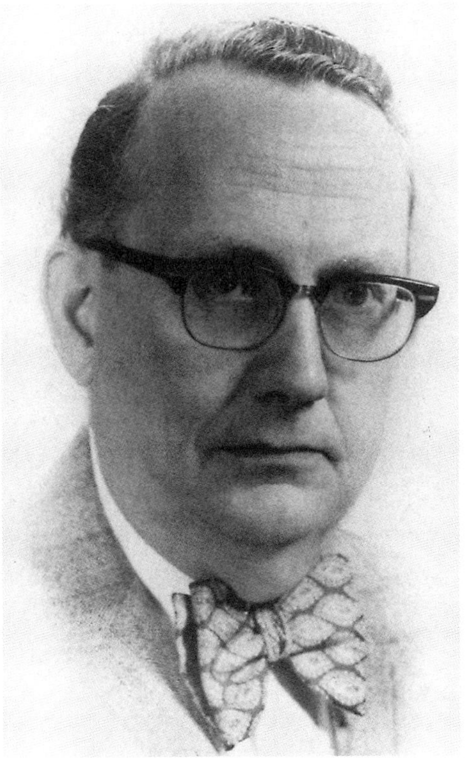

William M. Davis. Dr. Davis recalled in a 1996 interview that one of the most rewarding moments of his career was being selected "Teacher of the Year" after completing his term as City Chief of Staff in 1973.
Summa Health System

cation in those days. Basic science usually met Tuesday evenings and was preceded by 'study hall' at Little Joe's All Stars."

The Orthopaedic Education Committee also recommended that, in the Grad-4 year, each resident should have a six-month "elective" period of study at an institution of his own choosing. They also replaced the old case-presentation conference with an organized schedule of specific subjects to be presented at the Wednesday morning conference. Conferences are held daily throughout the week in 1998.

One recommendation, that City, General, and Children's Hospitals have one orthopaedic residency program, was not acceptable to the trustees of either adult hospital. "It became such a political push-pull situation," Dr. Hoyt said, "that we just forgot about it. The two programs get together for their educational activities, but they're administered separately to this day."

This was the sixties. That tumultuous era of sit-ins, "in your face" actions, and a prevailing "don't trust anyone over thirty" attitude. It is not surprising, therefore, that this meeting's minutes include the following:

"Dr. Walter Brown pointed out that the dress and appearance of the orthopaedic residents was deteriorating and suggested that new efforts be made along lines of professional appearance and neatness amongst the resident staff." The matter was referred to Buel Smith's teaching schedule committee, but he recalls "no great success in confronting this problem."

Then there were those little things that made the residents' lives a bit more bearable. This item from the August 12, 1969 meeting:

Bill Davis recalls that City's administration periodically went on a cost containment drive. Among its strictures, one paper napkin per tray going through the cafeteria line. More important from the residents' view, only one dessert per tray. "Carl Palechek [City, class of '67] solved the problem for all time by finger tasting all the desserts as he went down the cafeteria line. Administration withdrew under fire."

"A discussion was held on the state of morale of the House Staff in general and the problems this may produce in recruiting interns for the coming year. A letter from the Chief Resident lists several complaints on the part of the House Staff:

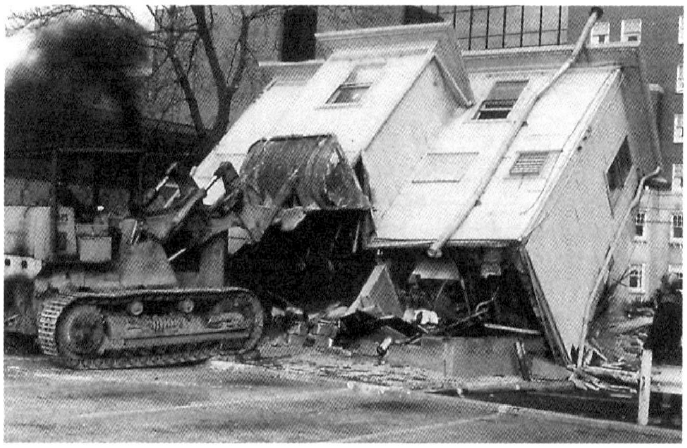

The Gray House, seen here being tipped over by a bulldozer, served as the residents' living quarters and occasional medical chart depository for many years before being demolished in 1980.

> The present system requiring payment for meals.
> Removal of the privilege of having families in the dining room on Sunday.
> Inadequate parking.
> Loss of the midnight snacks in the Gray House.

Staff members agreed that the residents had a valid case and, in time, the hospital made corrections.

Though City/Children's orthopaedic residency program underwent a major restructuring in 1969, its primary objective remained constant - teaching the practice of clinical medicine. Asked the department's mission, its Chairman, Pat Flanagan, once replied "quality patient care, education, and research. That's it - one, two, three. The patient comes first. You can't do education, the second one, without the first, the patient. And you do the third one (research) because you're doing the second."

Flanagan, one of the third generation of teachers and researchers in Akron orthopaedics, was a second year resident during City/Children's reorganization. In the twenty-three years since the program began in 1946, technological improvements and new procedures had poured out of major medical centers world-wide. Polio no longer dominated the summer months, thanks to the Salk and Sabin vaccines, successful replantation of severed limbs had become a reality, and emergency medicine had gone beyond the "snatch and grab" days. In this last case, Akron's orthopaedic residents and the Bath Township Fire and Rescue Squad played important roles. Moreover, in 1964, Akron's programs reached a turning point when the directors, Harry O'Dell and Walter Hoyt, brought their residents home for basic science and in so doing, developed an educational infrastructure locally. This would be an important factor in the 1970's when the programs finally achieved their long sought academic base: a medical school.

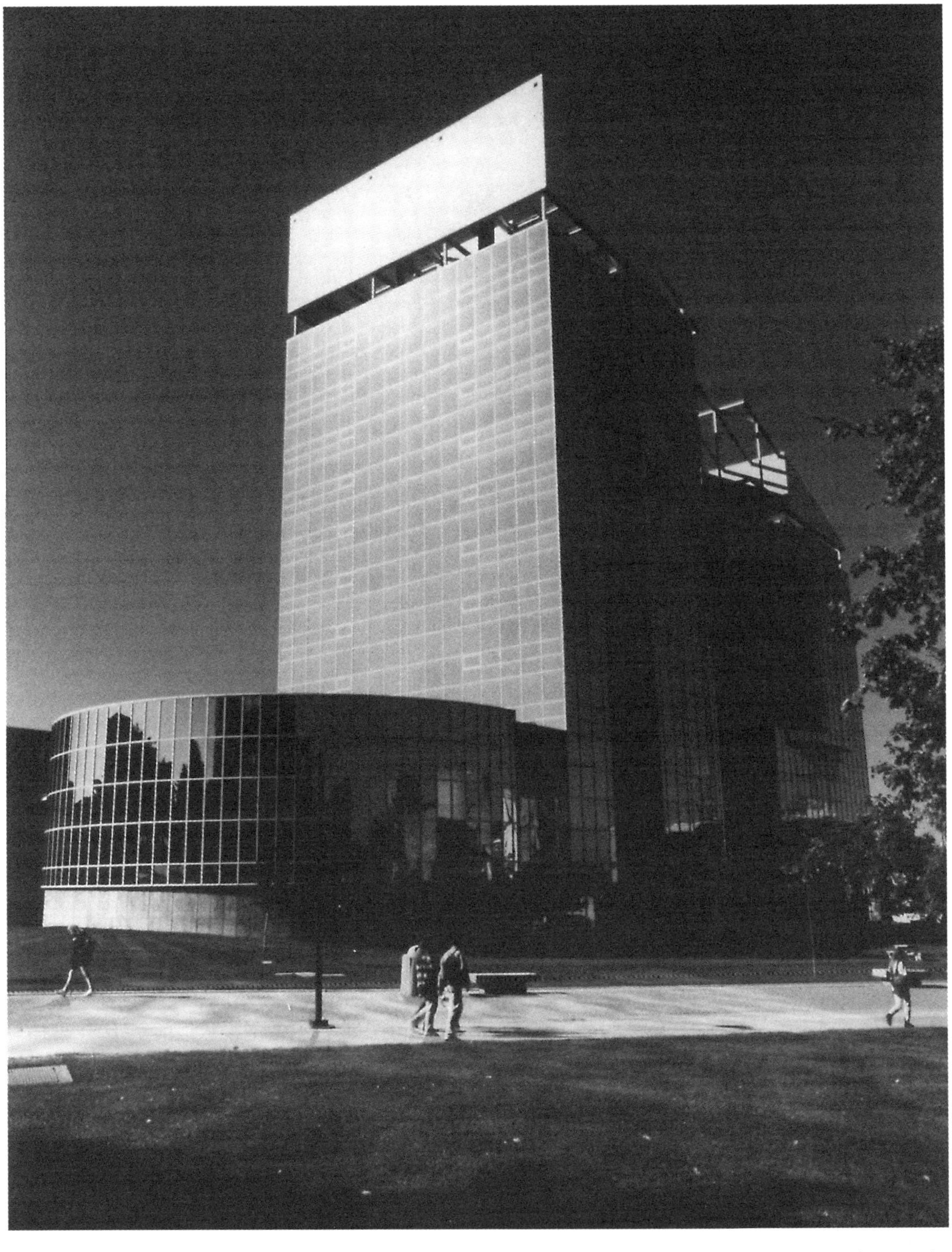

Polymer Science Building. This gleaming glass structure at the west end of the University of Akron's campus is home to the Department of Biomedical Engineering. **The University of Akron**

Chapter Three

1970-1982, Building An Academic Base

As the twentieth century rolled on toward its three-quarter mark, medical researchers around the world continued to build on earlier discoveries, improve orthopaedic technology, and turn theory into reality. For instance, physicians in Davos, Switzerland, produced new instruments, procedures, and hardware to treat fractures. England's Sir John Charnley, writing in Lancet in 1961, presented "Arthroplasty of the Hip: a new operation," which introduced hip replacement surgery. Knowledge increased, subspecialization evolved, and there was too much information to be taught in the existing residency program. This led to the first stirring of postresidency studies (fellowships) in orthopaedics. In Sweden, Carl Hirsch directed a postgraduate fellowship in the 1960's that stressed collaboration between clinicians and bioengineers, a collaboration that became commonplace in the 1970's and 1980's.

Knowledge of the musculoskeletal system and the skills developed to treat its ills had grown exponentially from the time of W.A. Hoyt, Sr., A.E. Davis, Fowler B. Roberts and the early days of Akron's orthopaedic residencies. In the 1970's, the second generation, men such as Harry O'Dell and Walter A. Hoyt, Jr., strengthened the residencies' educational infrastructure. Staff members did research, taught basic science, took time away from their practices to study under expert subspecialists, and learned new procedures, such as hip replacement surgery. When Northeastern Ohio Universities College of Medicine opened in 1977, Akron's orthopaedic surgeons were prepared and eager to make their contribution at this much needed academic base.

Meanwhile, advances in industrial technology brought grief to the Rubber City's tire industry, already reeling from management-labor conflicts and the struggle to maintain ancient plants. (No new tire factory had been built in Akron since the 1920's.) American automobiles, clunky, chrome studded, eight cylinder gas guzzlers, rolled along on pillow-soft bias ply tires. Enter the radial tire, a European product, fuel efficient, more costly, and more precisely produced than the bias ply. American manufacturers countered with the bias belted tire, but it was all for naught. Bias belted tires had 85 percent of the original equipment market share in 1971. Ten years later, bias belteds had 1 percent, radials, 99 percent. The resultant loss of jobs (Akron's factories were not refitted to make radials) devastated the city and its people. According to the authors of *Wheels of Fortune, A History of Rubber in Akron,*

There were fewer attending physicians in the seventies than there are today. Walter A. Hoyt, Jr., Edwin Mollin, and Zouhair Yassine comprised the group now known as Crystal Clinic, Inc. Buel Smith, Al Holderness, and Lynn Defreest had an office on Portage Trail in Cuyahoga Falls and serviced all the hospitals. James Roberts (Fowler B.'s son), Robert Clark, and George Mallo comprised a third group; Walter Brown, George Bischoff, and Adrian Davis a fourth. William Davis and James Parks practiced together for twenty-nine years, sharing experiences and coverage.

published by the *Akron Beacon Journal*, 1978 was the worst year: "When Firestone razed Plant 2, about $75,000 in property tax - about two-thirds of which benefitted Akron schools - was lost. And the city income tax lost as a result of the Firestone and Goodyear lay-offs totaled about $430,000....By the end of 1978, the profession that had defined Akron since early in the century - the building of car tires - was virtually gone."

Residents and Practitioners in the Early Seventies

Following their 1969 reorganization, City's orthopaedic staff pitched in and divided the work load. Robert Clark, Chief of the Service, ran the Division on a daily basis. George Mallo, City, class of '63, ran the hospital's amputation program. He also managed the residency program in the 1970s. Herb Thompson, City, class of '72, worked with him. Mallo and Thompson, partners since 1972, were team physicians at the University of Akron.

George Mallo, in charge of recruiting residents in the early seventies, recalled City's class of '74, Frank Forshew and Robert W. Patti. "A fractured pelvis delayed Dr. Forshew starting his residency. He'd had a year's internship here and then went into the Army. He called me from the service to say he was sending his X-rays. I can remember standing in the X-ray viewing room, looking at his fracture in the view box. I hired him, he came in a little late, finished his residency, and took a fellowship in hand surgery."

"Dr. Patti is from Akron," Mallo continued, "he took his internship out west. Before he finished his internship, he called me, came back here, interviewed, and took his residency at City." Dr. Patti practiced locally with Dr. Tom Bear and Dr. Flanagan, and now practices in Las Vegas."

According to Daniel Bethem, Patti became interested in non-operative management of low back pain while practicing in Akron. "He was Akron's first orthopaedic surgeon," Bethem said, "to become knowledgeable about all non-operative modalities. Not only physical therapy techniques, but also those 'treatments' outside the traditional spheres of orthopaedics such as chiropractic, massotherapy, and acupressure. His primary contributions were the initiation of McKenzie lumbar extension therapy for the treatment of lumbar disc disease and developing an understanding of sacroiliac dysfuntion."

Akron's second fellowship-trained hand surgeon, Frank C. Forshew, City, class of '74, divided his fellowship. Bill Davis recalls that "Dr. Forshew spent six months with Dr. Adrian E. Flatt at Iowa City and six months with Dr. Howard Kleinert in Louisville, Kentucky. He returned to Akron an accomplished hand and microvascular surgeon."

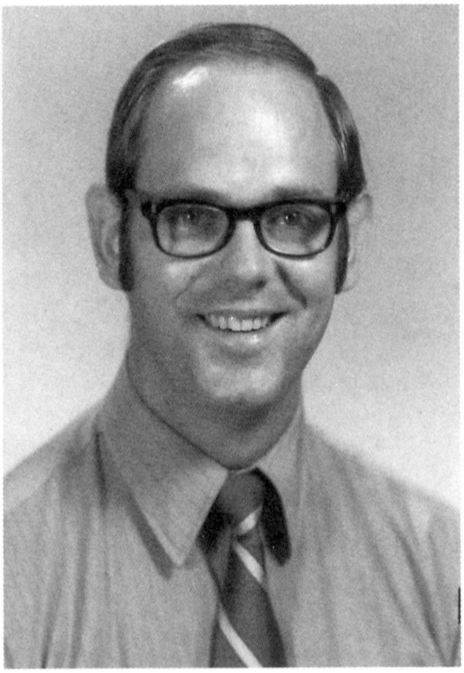

Frank Forshew. Dr. Forshew, shown here as a chief resident, took his fellowship under expert hand surgeons, Drs. Adrian E. Flatt and Howard Kleinert.

Replantation of severed limbs became technically feasible in the sixties. In the seventies, Jean Morton, R.N., had her "first experience with reattached parts," working with Dr. Forshew "on a young man who came from California to visit his grandmother and lost two fingers in a power lawn mower. Great nursing skill and patience were rewarded by successful replantation."

Speaking recently of replantation, Dr. Hoyt said, "this (microvascular surgery) is very sophisticated surgery. You have a fancy microscope and you have to suture arteries and nerves. It can take fifteen, twenty hours sometimes. The fact that it's being done here in Akron is an indication of the quality of the people who are here. People who are willing to take the time, learn the skills, and have the skill to do it. They get cases for replantation from all over the place because they have the capability of doing this difficult and time consuming surgery."

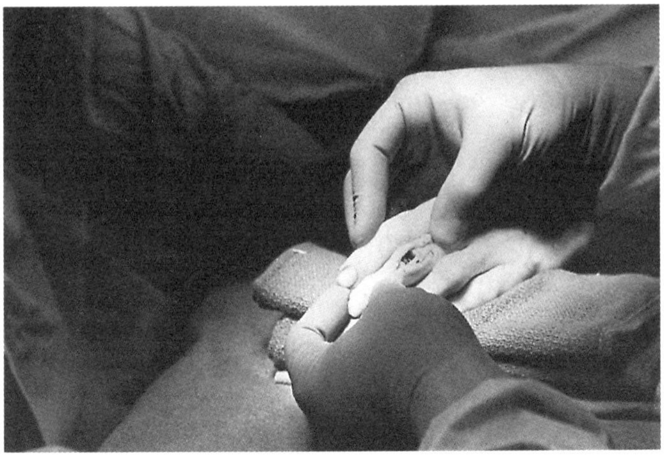

Dr. Frank Forshew's hands at work repairing the middle finger of the patient's left hand. **Summa Health System**

Bill Davis says that to his "best memory, Frank Forshew introduced microvascular technology in Akron. Dr. Forshew," Davis recalled, "revascularized an almost completely amputated arm on a patient from General Tire. I fixed the humerus that had been severed above the elbow and Frank repaired arteries, veins, and the major ner-

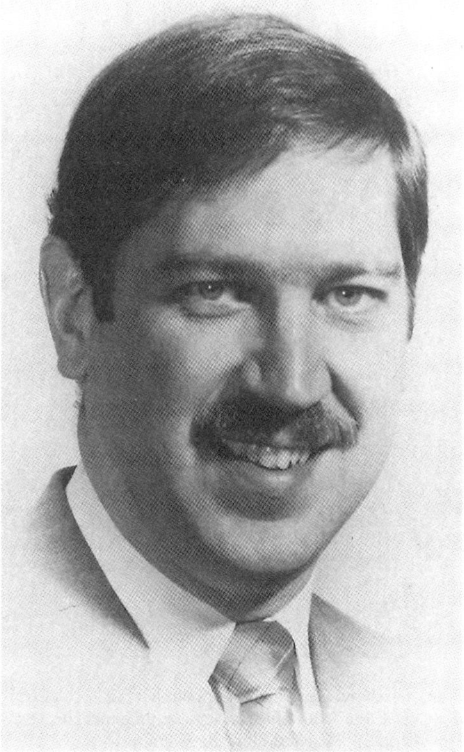

Thomas F. Bear was chief of staff at City Hospital in 1985.
Summa Health System

ves, except the ulnar nerve that had not been severed. The patient later returned to work with a good, functional extremity. To my memory," Davis concluded, "that was the first successful revascularization done in Akron." Dr. Forshew died in a plane crash in March 1992 while returning from a CME course on hand surgery held in Florida.

Akron's third generation orthopaedists started out practicing general orthopaedics, but, since the 1970's, subspecialization has brought many changes to their community practices. For example, Patrick Flanagan, Robert Patti, and Thomas Bear, City, classes of '73, '74, and '75 respectively, went into practice together in 1975. Recently, Bear recalled that he "did just about everything in pediatric orthopaedics but pelvic osteotomies and scoliosis surgery and, of course, no spina bifida surgery. But, beyond that, I took care of many other pediatric entities, cerebral palsy, or neurologically handicapped. I took care of patients with slipped capital femoral epiphysis, Perthes disease, pediatric trauma, pediatric fractures. But, during the twenty years I've been in practice, pediatric orthopaedic surgeons have come into town, set up practice, and the pediatric practice has gone into a more specialized field."

Adult orthopaedics has changed, too. When Bear hung out his shingle, he "did a lot of degenerative spine, a lot of laminectomies, and a lot of spinal fusions. I don't do spine any more because we now [1997] have five orthopaedic surgeons in town who limit their practice to spine. When I first went into practice there were two orthopaedic surgeons in town who did hand, Dr. William Davis and Dr. Thomas Reef. Counting the one plastic-surgeon-fellowship-trained, there are now nine hand surgeons here."

Over the years, Bear's community practice has taken on its own subspecialization. Today, he has a large arthroscopic practice, which evolved after the development of the arthroscope and the teaching of J. Whitaker Ewing, M.D., an American pioneer in arthroscopy. He also does knee reconstruction, joint replacement, and trauma. "Now," Bear said, "I still do a fair amount of shoulder surgery, but there are four men who essentially limit their practice to shoulder. We have several fellowship trained total joint surgeons, hip and knee here in Akron, whereas when I started in practice, there were none. I still do a lot of total joints."

Interest in orthopaedics among medical students has increased tremendously over the last quarter century. Pat Flanagan recalls that when he was an intern, "looking for an orthopaedic residency [in the late sixties], there were few applicants. Following the development of total joints and arthroscopy in the early seventies, the number of individuals interested in orthopaedics continued to increase to the level it is today."

"The technique of arthroscopy [in Akron] was pioneered by Dr. Whit Ewing, along with George Mallo and Herb Thompson," Flanagan continued. "Although Ewing had no fellowship training, he developed the science of arthroscopy to the point where he was able to pass on his knowledge to others. At one point, when he was a second year resident, he told me, 'if I'm ever going to look into a knee joint, I'm going to do it with my eyeball, not a scope.' I've reminded him of that on multiple occasions and he says, 'it just shows how wrong you can be.'" In arthroscopy's early days, the clinician looked into an extremely bright light, bright enough to damage the retina. Now, he or she watches a television monitor. "Dr. Ewing enjoyed a strong referral base from all members of the local community and would perform up to a dozen arthroscopies a day, and the development of surgical procedures through the arthroscope has steadily increased," Flanagan concluded.

Administrative Changes

City's orthopaedic division became a department in 1971. The benefits were great - and deserved. "We were a section in the department of surgery," Dr. Hoyt recalled. "Achieving departmental status meant we sat on the hospital executive committee. We had total responsibility for our own staff. We could appoint men to our staff and we controlled our budget rather than having to go through general surgery. And, we had total control over our residency program and our orthopaedic beds. Orthopaedics had come of age and departmental status was well justified on the basis of volume of surgery performed, number of beds occupied, extent of research undertaken, and the quality of the members of the orthopaedic staff." Three residents were admitted to City's program each year after departmental status was achieved.

Across town, Akron General Hospital was in the throes of a building program in the late sixties and its main entrance shifted once again, from Wabash Avenue to Codding Street when the 100 Building opened. The hospital became Akron General Medical Center in 1973. In 1975, Buel Smith succeeded Harry O'Dell as Chairman of AGMC's Department of Orthopaedic Surgery.

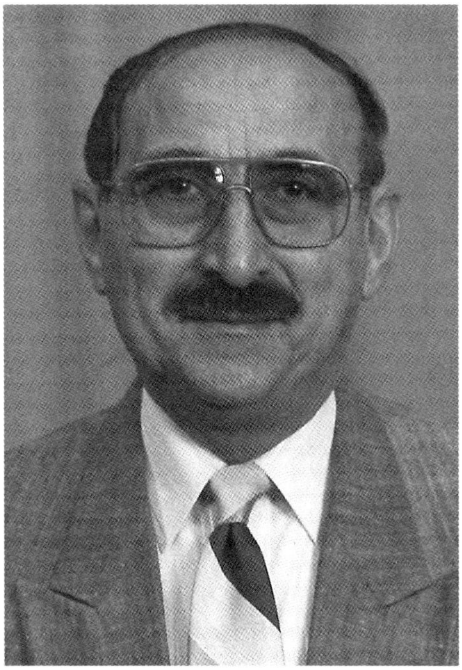

Zouhair C. Yassine. Dr. Yassine has devoted hundreds of hours teaching anatomy to NEOUCOM freshmen and in May 1996 he received the Dean's Award in recognition of his contributions to the medical school.
Summa Health System

"Bring Backs" Continue

Michael J. Askew, Ph.D., Director of the Walter A. Hoyt, Jr. Musculoskeletal Laboratory, says that Akron's orthopaedic surgeons "have been in the forefront in bringing advances into clinical practice in the treatment of bone and joint infections, joint replacement surgery, arthroscopy, and hand and microvascular surgery with orthopaedic applications." He cites Drs. Hoyt, Sr., A.E. Davis, and Van Buren for their work with sulfathiazole in the treatment of osteomyelitis and other bone infections.

Local orthopaedists have been bringing home new procedures and equipment since Fowler B. Roberts, who did some early scoliosis work, brought the Risser operating table to Akron. Zouhair C. Yassine, M.D. City, class of '56, introduced his colleagues to the Swiss method of ORIF [open reduction, internal fixation] in the early 1970s. Dr. Yassine recalls that, in the 1950s and 1960s, "the accepted philosophy was that the more comminuted the intraarticular fracture (such as the elbow and the knee), the less was the indication for open reduction as the tools to properly internally fix them were not available. Olecranon fractures were treated with the long half threaded flexible Leimbach screw, which broke more often than not. Hip fractures were treated by Smith Peterson nails, with and without Thornton plates or the Jewett nail, the angle of which could be manually changed by a strong resident. Not uncommonly, they broke at the junction of the nail and the plate. Comminuted long bone shaft fractures were treated by skeletal traction followed by cast immobilization after evidence of some callus formation."

Meanwhile, researchers in the ski resort town of Davos, Switzerland, were making great advances in treating fractures by internal fixation. The dominant principle of the ASIF (Association for the Study of Internal Fixation) and the AO (Association for Osteosynthesis), according to Dr. Yassine, "was to avoid the so-called 'cast disease,' with its muscle atrophy, joint stiffness, and bony osteoporosis, which often results from prolonged cast immobilization."

Yassine attended an instructional course in Davos in 1969 and was tremendously impressed. The Swiss, he said, "devised techniques in compressing fractures, solidly fixing them together, thus eliminating the need for casting and allowing early mobilization and weight bearing. They devised plates and screws of all shapes and sizes to fix bones as long as a femur and as small as a phalanx. They differentiated between hypertrophic and atrophic pseudoarthroses and recommended variations of the proper treatment in each case. They emphasized the importance of tackling the distal fibula first in treating ankle fractures. Treatment of patellar and olecranon fractures with K wire fixation reinforced with cerclage wires permitted immediate mobilization without plaster fixation."

In Akron, hospital administrators at first refused to purchase the Swiss instrumentation sets. They considered the Davos methods, Dr. Yassine said, "too revolutionary, not the accepted standard in Akron, or the United States." Yassine decided that good results would win the day. He convinced his colleagues to buy the sets and let him treat their cases, and his, according to the Swiss AO techniques. He dragged the heavy bags of instruments from hospital to hospital, developing a brachial plexus stretch paresthesia in the process. His pains were rewarded when Saturday after Saturday at the morning fracture conferences, he presented cases showing good results. By this time, many American orthopaedists had been to Davos and the AO technique was spreading rapidly through the United States. The hospitals gave in, purchasing all the appropriate instrument sets and the AO principles and techniques became accepted methods of treating fractures in Akron.

Hip replacement surgery, a very important "bring-back," came to Akron in 1971. In orthopaedics, metal plates have been used for internal fixation of fractured bones since 1886. "But," Dr. Askew says, "performance of these and other metal implants was greatly enhanced by the introduction of low carbon stainless steels and the introduction (by Venable and Stuck in 1936) of the cobalt chrome alloy known as vitallium."

After the Second World War, the Judet brothers, French researchers, became interested in materials for implants and began investigating an acrylic hip replacement in 1946. They introduced an endo-prosthesis of nylon for replacement of the femoral head in high neck fractures in 1949. F.R. Thompson, writing in the *New York Journal of Medicine,* presented his "Vitallium intramedullary hip prosthesis" in 1952.

In 1959, England's Sir John Charnley began investigating a variety of materials, Dr. Askew said, "including polytetrafluoroethylene ("Teflon") for use in joint replacements. In 1968, Charnley presented the world with the modern day joint arthroplasty incorporating metal and polyethylene components fixed in place with polymethylmethacrylate bone cement."

Total hip replacement and total knee replacement entered the scene in Akron in the seventies and required special training. Just as early general surgeons apprenticed themselves to an outstanding orthopaedic surgeon, orthopaedists now searched out the best hand surgeon, the top spine surgeon, and learned from them. Walter A. Hoyt, Jr. studied under Dr. Frank Stinchfield in New York and performed the first total hip replacement in Akron in 1971. Buel Smith and Harry O'Dell established the protocols at Akron General Hospital for total knee and total hip surgery in 1972. Dr. Smith took special training in these procedures with John Charnley at Wrightington Hospital in England, Dr. O'Dell at the Mayo Clinic.

Charnley's work had other applications, too, according to Dr. Askew. "The work of Gunston, Insall, and Walker in the design of knee replacements, and the emergence of the science of biomaterials, not perhaps from its birthplaces, but at least from its nurseries, Clemson, South Carolina, and New Orleans, Louisiana, owe much to the success of the dedicated, conscientious work of Sir John Charnley."

Harry O'Dell recalls that, in the seventies, "patients for total knee or total hip were admitted on Sunday and were not operated on until Friday. Because of the fear of infection, these patients were isolated in a private room and anybody visiting them had to wear a gown and mask. At the time of surgery, the nurses, the anesthesiologists, the orthopaedic residents, and staff members gowned in a separate room and actually walked on special carpet into the operating room. There they wore special clothes for the procedure."

Bill Davis recalls banning flowers in the patient's room, especially potted plants because of the soil bacteria. "We were terribly, terribly afraid of infection," he said, "which in a total joint, would have been an absolute catastrophe."

Orthopaedic surgeons were not the only ones learning these new procedures. Jean Morton, RN, head nurse on City's 3-east at the time, recalls that the hospital "sent me to Minneapolis when we started to do total hip replacements. I was there for a week along with nurses from all over the United States. It was like a new world opening."

Subspecialization Comes to Akron

As the seventies began, the rapid development of subspecialization caused concern among Fellows of the American Academy of Orthopaedic Surgeons. They worried about their specialty splintering into separate academies, each giving its own Board examinations. And, realizing that subspecialization was here to stay, they worried about the educational quality of these "fellowships" that were the primary method of teaching subspecialties.

Subspecialization was a hot, worrisome topic when Philip D. Wilson, Jr., M.D., (son of the physician who organized the American Hospital in Oxford, England in 1942) gave his Presidential Address to the American

Academy of Orthopaedic Surgeons in 1973. Academy Fellows had complained to Wilson about subspecialty satellite organizations and meetings that had grown up around the AAOS's annual gathering. (The senior Academy Fellows perhaps forgot that some forty years earlier, as brash young orthopaedists searching for a place to meet, discuss problems, and seek solutions, they had similarly discomfited the august American Orthopaedic Association.)

Having characterized the Academy's annual meeting as "a forum of educational interchange," Wilson went on to say that subspecialization, or as he preferred, "supraspecialization" [indicating an added skill], was simply continuing medical education -- the Academy's cornerstone. Furthermore, these supraspecialists "who, by extra added study and experience develop greater proficiency than our colleagues in one area of orthopaedics, have acquired a special area of expertise. The supraspecialist is entitled to something more because he has worked for it."

Wilson then speculated about how those "who have been left behind in this one particular concentrated area of orthopaedics" would react to supraspecialization. "Some of us," Wilson said, "will resume our education [and] acquire this new knowledge, whereupon we also are entitled to join the experts in its use for the benefit of our patients. Others will be content to be informed about it, so that we may refer our patients when such new knowledge is applicable to their problem. Still others, through unfortunate isolation, never become informed of the new knowledge in the first place. This leads us to commit an error of omission when we fail to direct a patient with a suitable indication to a source where he may benefit. Another group of us, however, rush to use the new knowledge without going to the trouble of mastering the science behind it. This group commits the most grievous error of all, for they risk the well-being of their patients unjustifiably."

The real question for Wilson was how to integrate the subspecialties into the Academy and he charged the supraspecialist "to make his new knowledge freely available as soon as possible to other competent orthopaedic surgeons." If there are valid reasons for restricting use of a new technique, "the knowledge of it should not be repressed, but should be fully exposed where all aspects of it may be examined, rejected, or accepted."

Furthermore, Wilson thought it "not illogical for supraspecialists to band together in separate societies, clubs, associations. But, I also charge them with the responsibility for bringing back their expertise to the rest of us, to the whole specialty, so that as many patients as possible may benefit." Today, subspecialty organizations abound, but the Academy escaped fragmentation. "We dodged a pretty big bullet," W.A. Hoyt, Jr. recalled.

Dr. Wilson addressed the American Academy of Orthopaedic Surgeons

Bill Davis came to his subspecialty "of necessity." Twinsburg's Chrysler stamping plant was sending an average of ten serious hand cases per week to his service at City Hospital. He was a bootstrap subspecialist (not fellowship trained) whose first teacher, in 1947, was the master hand surgeon, Sterling Bunnell. "I hated every minute of those Tuesday afternoons at Letterman General Hospital when I had to scrub with Sterling Bunnell," Davis recalled. "Bunnell was so meticulous, nobody wanted to scrub with him. As it turned out, it was the best two months of Tuesday afternoons I ever spent."

at a time of rapidly growing interest in subspecialty postgraduate education (fellowships). This popularity brought questions about the fellowships' educational quality. At the time, program quality depended solely on the integrity of the orthopaedist directing the fellowship.

W.A. Hoyt, Jr. recalls that, while the Residency Review Committee for Orthopaedics [the RRC] monitored residency programs, "there was no quality control over postgraduate study. The fellowship director issued his own certificate saying, for example, 'the Fellow spent a year here and did nothing but arthroscopy.' Now, he may have been in the director's basement looking through old records. That wasn't doing arthroscopy."

Two strong committees have monitored the programs since the seventies. One, the AMA's Accreditation Council for Graduate Medical Education [ACGME] and its Residency Review Committees [RRC], are the accrediting bodies for training programs. The Academy formed the Advisory Council for Orthopaedic Resident Education, or ACORE. ACORE members made a list of those orthopaedists giving fellowships, classified them as to subspecialty, established performance standards, and published a book, *Postgraduate Orthopaedic Fellowships.* According to the 1995 AAOS edition (ACORE published the first nine editions), the Residency Review Committee for Orthopaedics "currently provides accreditation of orthopaedic fellowships in seven categories: Adult Reconstructive Orthopaedics, Hand Surgery, Musculoskeletal Oncology, Orthopaedic Sports Medicine, Orthopaedic Surgery of the Spine, Orthopaedic Trauma, Pediatric Orthopaedics."

Beginning in the late sixties, many Akron orthopaedists went away to study under orthopaedists who were leaders in their respective subspecialties. Ivan Gradisar went to Case Western Reserve to study biomechanical research under Albert H. Burstein, Ph.D. Robert Bell studied the shoulder under Rich Hawkins, M.D. in London, Ontario, Canada. Daniel Bethem studied the spine at the Twin Cities Scoliosis Center at the University of Minnesota. Barry Greenberg received specialized training in rehabilitation at Rancho Los Amigos Rehabilitation Hospital in California. Walter Hoyt, Jr. studied hip replacement surgery under Frank Stinchfield, M.D. at Columbia University.

Harry O'Dell studied hip replacement at the Mayo Clinic. Buel Smith went to the source, studying hip replacement surgery with Sir John Charnley in England.

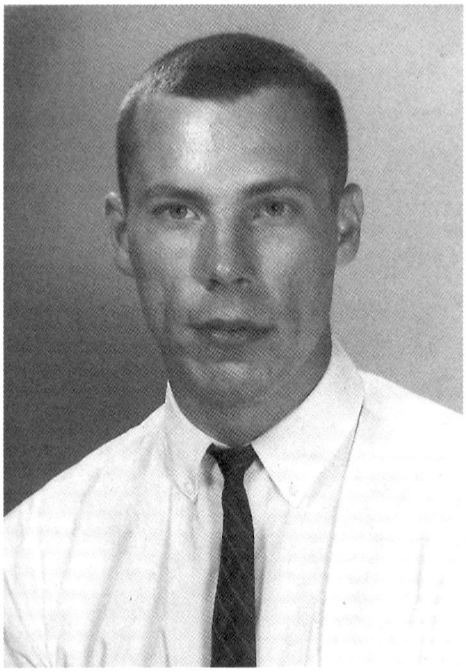

Thomas C. Reef. Dr. Reef was Akron's first fellowship trained hand surgeon in 1970. **Summa Health System**

City Hospital's hand service, established on January 2, 1972, as a joint venture of orthopaedic and plastic surgery, represents the first formal recognition of an orthopaedic subspecialty in Akron. Appointed chief of the service, Bill Davis served for two years. "There was a question of who was going to do hands," he recalled. "We set up a program at City in which the plastic surgeons had one-sixth of the emergency referrals and orthopaedics, the remainder. Then we set up the requirement that, in future, anyone heading the hand service would be fellowship trained."

Two years later, Thomas C. Reef, M.D., City, class of '66, Akron's first fellowship-trained orthopaedic surgeon, headed the hand service. Later, Dr. Reef was chief of hand surgery at both City and Akron General. In May, 1975, the hospital's Medical Executive Committee approved the following qualifications to practice hand surgery. "1. Board certified Ortho[paedic Surgery], PLS [Plastic Surgery], General Surgery. 2. Consecutive one year fellowship. 3.Physician's practice limited to hand surgery. Ten months to be covered by 'Hand Service.' Two months to be covered by 'Plastics' -plastic surgeons who had adequate training and experience in hand surgery as determined by the Chief of Hand Service." According to Walter Hoyt, Jr., "these are stringent requirements, but essential, to assure quality."

As part of the 1969 reorganization, Akron's orthopaedic residents were encouraged to take a three to six months elective at academic centers across the country. They learned a lot about subspecialization, they worked with academicians, and they brought back new techniques and procedures.

In the 1970's, when subspecialist education was in its infancy, nine Akron orthopaedic residents took fellowships. They include: Charles Bellitti (hand), Daniel Bethem (spine), Frank Forshew (hand), Ivan Gradisar (research), Barry Greenberg (spine), Patrick T. Hergenroeder (hand and sports medicine), John F. Krempen (spine), Tom Reef (hand), Dennis S. Weiner (pediatric orthopaedics). Bellitti, Hergenroeder, and Krempen, all Akron General Medical Center alumni, practice elsewhere; two City alumni, Forshew and

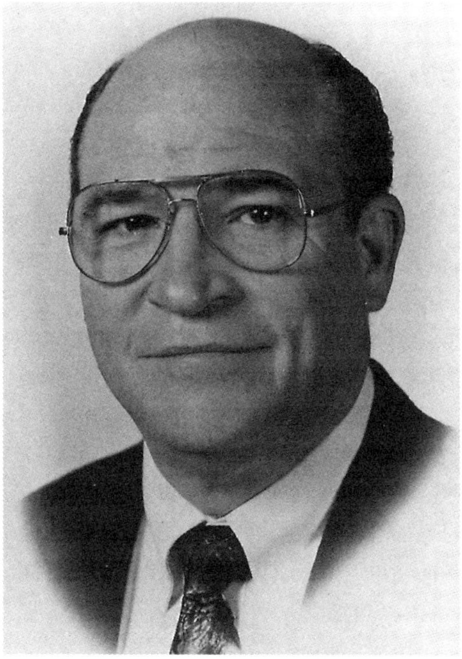

Barry J. Greenberg. As a fourth year resident at Akron General Medical Center, Dr. Greenberg studied with pioneers in spinal surgery at Rancho Los Amigos Hospital. He also served as chief of staff at City Hospital in 1991.

Reef, are deceased, Bethem [City] retired in 1996, Gradisar [City], Greenberg [AGMC], and Weiner [AGMC] practice in Akron.

Barry J. Greenberg, Akron General, class of '72, took his six-month elective course in 1971 at Rancho Los Amigos Rehabilitation Hospital in Downey, California. According to Daniel Bethem, Rancho Los Amigos was "one of the premier spinal surgery institutions in the country in the early seventies. Jacqueline Perry had just instituted the use of the halo. Mark Hoffer, Charles Bonnett, and John Brown were in the forefront of the treatment of scoliosis. Shannon Stauffer had just begun his work in spinal trauma, and Vert Mooney had a low back pain unit at the institution. Barry Greenberg was trained by all of these." Greenberg presented "Halo-Femoral Distraction and Posterior Spinal Fusion for Paralytic Scoliosis" at the Sixth Scoliosis Research Society meeting in the Fall of 1971.

While at Rancho Los Amigos, Barry Greenberg made the acquaintance of Mark Yanke, a certified prosthetist and orthotist. According to Dan Bethem, "Greenberg and Yanke developed the Akron version of a thoraco-lumbosacral orthosis for scoliosis which obviated the circumferential constriction and its complication of rib cage deformity and callus formation of the anterosuperior iliac spine. The Akron T.L.S.O. provided a means for non-operative treatment of scoliosis when diagnosed during its early stages," Bethem concluded.

Daniel Bethem, City, class of '77, took a one year fellowship in spine at the Twin Cities Scoliosis Center in 1978, returned to Akron and limited his practice to spinal disorders. He was the first orthopaedic surgeon in Akron to limit his practice to the subspecialty of spine surgery. Bethem studied under four presidents of the Scoliosis Research Society while at the Center: John Moe, Robert Winter, David Bradford, and John Lonstein.

Bethem's return brought his Twin Cities' teachers' influence to help children with scoliosis. "John Moe was now present in Akron," Bethem says, "in that facet fusions with wide lateral posterior fusions were performed for scoliosis. Triplanar correction of spinal deformities became surgical goals that were achieved by contouring of Harrington rods utilizing both distraction and compression. Combined anterior and posterior spinal surgery became commonplace in the treatment of severe deformities. Risser casting techniques, created at the Twin Cities Scoliosis Center, were utilized to provide not only improved fit, but also improved patient comfort and mobility with greater correction." Postoperative bracing replaced Risser casts in 1983, and in 1985, Bethem introduced segmental spinal fixation here, which eliminated postoperative immobilization.

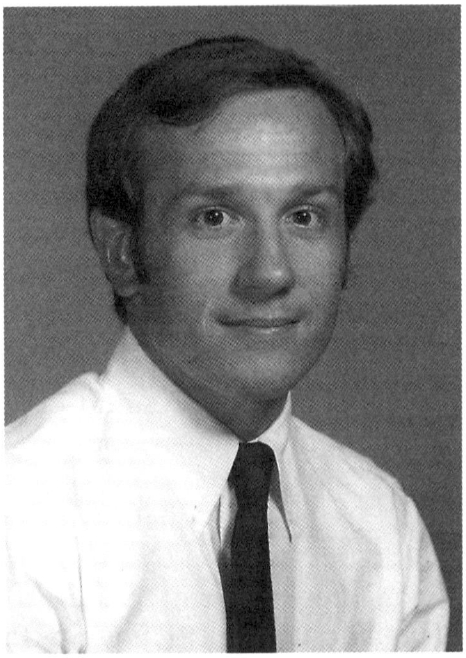

Daniel Bethem. Dr. Bethem was Akron's first subspecialist in spinal surgery. In 1978 he was a recipient of the Moe Scoliosis Fellowship in Minneapolis.
Summa Health System

Scoliosis remains a serious orthopaedic problem. Dennis S. Weiner, Akron General, class of '69, recalls that he and Barry Greenberg "developed the first scoliosis screening program ever done in this area. It was one of two pilot projects in the State of Ohio under the auspices of the Bureau of Crippled Children's Services. The first year we screened 28,000 sixth, seventh, and eighth graders in city, county, and parochial schools and identified over 2,000 positive cases." Scoliosis screening is done throughout the state today and, according to Dr. Weiner, "the numbers [of afflicted children] are about the same."

Pediatric orthopaedics was not officially recognized as a subspecialty until the late seventies, several years after Weiner completed his residency. "There weren't formal fellowships available [in 1970]," he recalled, "so I had to design my own, spending eighteen months travelling around North America." Weiner studied spinal disorders with Dr. Ian McNab at the Wellesley Hospital in Toronto and with Dr. John Hall at Sick Children's Hospital, also in Toronto. He also spent periods of time at Rancho Los Amigos, where Barry Greenberg would study also, Sonoma State Hospital, at Stanford University working with Dr. Eugene Bleck, and at Newington, Connecticut, Children's Hospital.

While training with Ian McNab, Weiner wrote the first paper on the use of chymopapain on thirty-two patients in the *Canadian Journal of Surgery*. On returning home, he began extensive research into many pediatric orthopaedic problems. According to Michael Askew, "Dr. Weiner is a continuing force in research done by the orthopaedic residents." Since 1975, research at Children's into pediatric orthopaedic conditions has resulted in nearly one hundred publications, including a book on Pediatric Orthopaedics.

Orthotics (braces), prosthetics (artificial limbs), and rehabilitation (restoring function) form an important triad in orthopaedics. Orthotics came to the Rubber City in the twenties and thirties and consisted mainly of bracing for pediatric problems. "When poliomyelitis became rampant," Dr. Hoyt said "there was a need for an unusually large number of braces of all types. At the time, Bart Crowley was the only orthotist in Akron. In addition, Joe Yanke, [Mark Yanke's father] came from Cleveland and attended our clinics on a weekly basis, sharing with Bart Crowley the responsibility of providing braces for the clinic patients. Ben Rivlin, an orthopaedic shoe man, came down from Cleveland in the fifties and provided the orthopaedic shoe." Mr. Crowley's Akron Brace Company, long a West Market Street fixture, closed some years ago.

Today, top quality prosthetists and orthotists at Akron Orthotic Solutions, Novacare Orthotics and Prosthetics, and Yanke Bionics serve the Akron area. Norm Shamp, a bi-lateral amputee, came to Akron from Cleveland to found Shamp Prosthetic-Orthotic Service, which is now Novacare.

A Non-Traditional Medical School

Akron's orthopaedic residencies seemed to be developing satisfactorily by the mid-seventies, but, in the long term, their future remained doubtful. They needed the academic support a medical school provided. It was the old refrain, heard since 1946: "All you have," as Walter A. Hoyt, Jr. recalled, "is a bunch of well-trained, aggressive orthopaedic surgeons doing the teaching. The academic environment is lacking."

Finally, the residencies obtained their academic base with the opening of the Northeastern Ohio Universities College of Medicine in September 1977. NEOUCOM, founded on November 26, 1973, was a new kind of medical school, developed according to the MEDCO plan, first advanced by Dr. Milton Eisenhower, former president of Johns Hopkins University and brother of U.S. President Dwight Eisenhower. NEOUCOM is a consortium of the three nearby state universities - the University of Akron, Kent State University, and Youngstown State University. By relying on these institutions and on nearby community hospitals, by creating a six-year B.S.--M.D. curriculum, and by having many practicing physicians donate their time as teachers, NEOUCOM operates at a lower cost than a traditional medical school.

Stanley W. Olson, M.D., the new medical school's Chief Executive Officer, faced a herculean organizational task, according to Buel Smith. "In the months following his appointment," Smith said, "Dr. Olson had to recruit a faculty, plan a six-year curriculum, establish standards for admission, secure

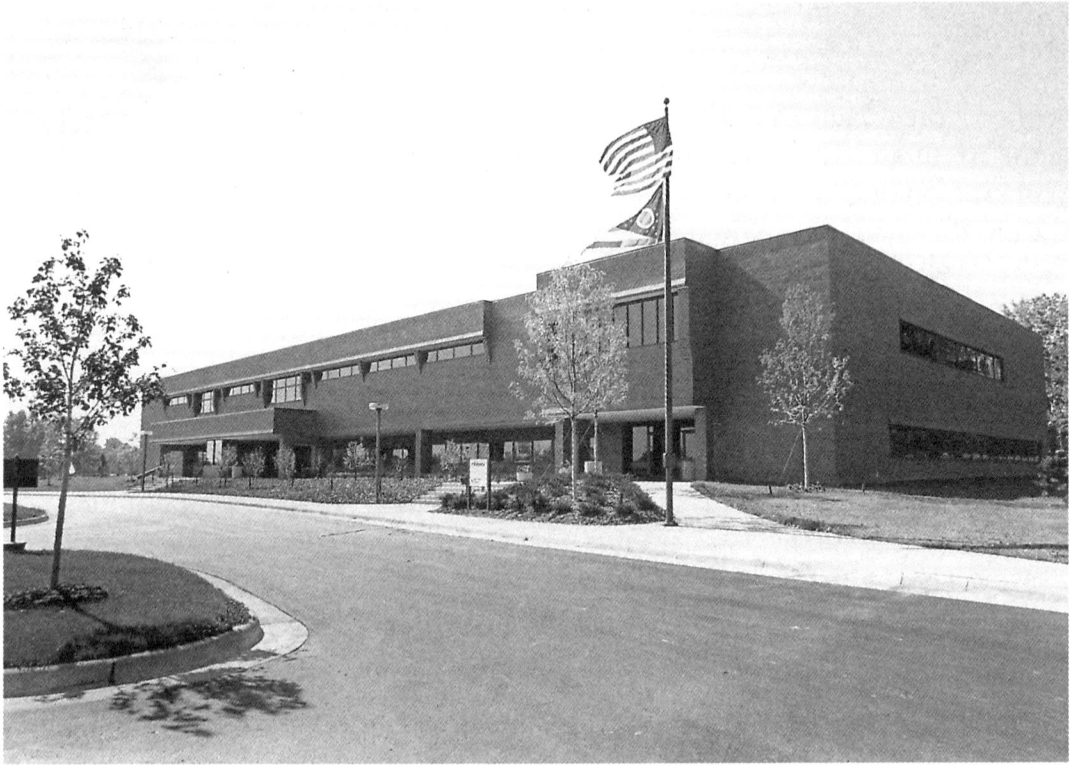

NEOUCOM. Since 1977 area physicians have donated their time to educate their successors.
Northeastern Ohio Universities College of Medicine

association agreements with the hospitals, plan a campus, and seek accreditation by the Liaison Committee on Medical Education. Incredibly, Dr. Olson accomplished each one of these goals."

The new medical school attracted a great deal of attention within the profession; 750 people applied for 42 available positions in Phase 1 of the B.S.-M.D. program for 1975-76. Robert A. Liebelt, M.D. was appointed Dean and Professor of Anatomy in July 1974. A Council of Chiefs (Chiefs in each clinical specialty at the various hospitals) was established. Dean Liebelt and the Trustees then designated one of the Chiefs as Chairman of the Council. Walter A. Hoyt, Jr., M.D., was the first Chairman of the Council of Chiefs of Orthopaedic Surgery, appointed on May 6, 1975, serving until 1982.

Akron's orthopaedic surgeons have contributed their time and talents to NEOUCOM from the beginning. Dennis S. Weiner, Chairman of Children's Hospital's Department of Orthopaedic Surgery, recalls that "Walt Hoyt was intensely involved in the medical school. He chaired the musculoskeletal curriculum committee composed of myself, Drs. Patrick Flanagan, and Buel Smith. Other orthopaedists were involved, too, in drawing up the curriculum, which took two years to do."

Dr. Hoyt says "we needed this academic base. Stan Olson was the lead man with the medical school and Bob Liebelt was the Dean. Four or five of us spent hundreds of hours working with those two men developing the framework upon which the whole academic curriculum is built. When the time came to obtain final accreditation, Dean Liebelt came to me and said, 'Hoyt, you know more about this place than anyone else. I want you to chair the committee that will get us final accreditation from the AMA." It was a daunting task. "We produced a 3,000 page report on the organization and entire structure of the medical school. The AMA came here, spent three days inspecting the facility, and gave us full accreditation in March 1981."

Besides providing the long sought academic credentials, the medical school gave orthopaedists the opportunity to teach first year medical students. Dr. Norman Taslitz, Chairman of NEOUCOM's Anatomy Department, welcomed their involvement as well as that of clinicians from other specialties. Dr. Hoyt recalled that "Dr. Weiner taught pediatric orthopaedics as a specialty; Dr. Yassine taught anatomy. Dr. Buel Smith was actively involved; a number of men were. They made rounds with the medical students, had sit-down conferences in orthopaedic surgery."

Dr. Yassine says that "the orthopaedic residency programs at Akron City and Akron General Hospitals were quick to offer orthopaedic rotations in M-3 and orthopaedic electives for the M-4 students. In addition, we felt we should be involved at the M-1 level, specifically in anatomy because the presence of one orthopaedist with whom the students could identify would be of great help when dissecting and studying the musculoskeletal system." And so it was that Dr. Yassine began spending two afternoons a week in the dissecting laboratory, "going from table to table answering questions, quizzing students on subjects already learned."

Moreover, City's and General's orthopaedic department chairmen have always encouraged their residents to attend these dissection sections. Buel Smith says that the residents "participated in the anatomy course, presenting lectures and assisting in the laboratory instruction of the musculoskeletal system, and were repeatedly commended by the professor of anatomy." The chairmen also recruit enough staff orthopaedists to offer the students sessions on "surface anatomy" of the upper and lower extremities. Dr. Smith recalls that, in the early years, "the M-4 year was devoted largely to electives and the Council of Orthopaedic Surgery offered electives in orthopaedics, sports medicine, pediatric orthopaedics, orthopaedic oncology, and other electives designed by the individual student. Fellowships in orthopaedic research were also offered, especially during the summer months. As a combination, these electives provided many students with additional introduction to the anatomy, physical diagnosis, and treatment of the musculoskeletal system."

And so, academic medicine, in the form of NEOUCOM, came to the Rubber City. According to Buel Smith, the Northeastern Ohio Universities College of Medicine met a "clearly defined need for physicians in this part of

Ohio." NEOUCOM, Smith says, "was essential to guarantee the continued progress of the residencies in orthopaedic surgery. In return, the orthopaedic surgeons, both faculty and residents, have made a significant contribution to the College."

Research in Biomechanics Comes to Akron

Academic support for the residency programs was strengthened still further by the development in the late 1970s of collaboration between the orthopaedists at City Hospital and the engineers of the University of Akron. This collaboration had its origins outside the city, in the larger medical community to which the Akron programs had always been closely tied.Its inspiration lay in Sweden where, in the 1960s, an orthopaedic surgeon named Carl Hirsch had established a significant fellowship, one that stressed collaboration between the clinician and the academician. According to Michael Askew, Ph.D, Hirsch's fellowship "exposed orthopaedic surgeons to a research experience and set the stage for the explosion of academic biomechanics in the seventies and eighties. This fellowship attracted many young surgeons from around the world, including Victor Frankel, M.D. of New York.

On returning from his fellowship, Frankel began collaborating on biomechanical research with applications to orthopaedic surgery with a Ph.D. student at Brooklyn Polytechnic Institute, Albert H. Burstein." Askew regards the pair as modern medical explorers. "Dr. Frankel's twentieth century partnership with Dr. Burstein was to orthopaedic biomechanics in the United States as the settlement of the Jamestown colony in the seventeenth century had been to the nation itself."

The Frankel-Burstein collaboration took place first in New York, then at Case Western Reserve University in Cleveland, Ohio. They produced numerous landmark papers and, in 1970, the influential textbook, *Orthopaedic Biomechanics*. But, Dr. Askew believes that the greatest contribution of Frankel and Burstein was that, "as a team, they demonstrated the benefits of collaboration between clinicians and engineer/scientists, and were the prototype of such collaboration."

Particularly because Frankel and Burstein were so close to Akron, their collaboration affected the Rubber City's orthopaedic residencies. Ivan A. Gradisar, Jr., City's second fellowship-trained orthopaedic surgeon, took his fellowship in bioengineering with Albert Burstein at Cleveland's Case Western Reserve University in 1973. He joined the teaching staff at City Hospital after his training and, Gradisar said "began collaborative research projects, supported by the National Institutes of Health, with the University of Akron's Department of Mechanical Engineering on a non-invasive acoustic technique for the detection of joint arthritis." Gradisar recalls that "up to that

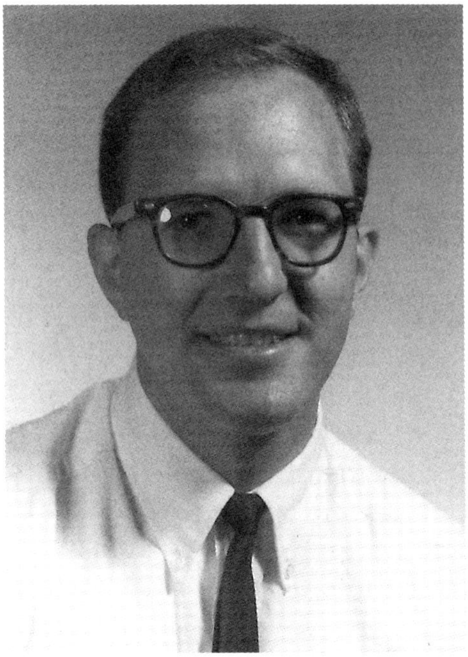

Ivan A. Gradisar, Jr. has served for many years as Medical Director of Research at Summa's Department of Orthopaedics. Dr. Gradisar is the only one of his colleagues to have taken a fellowship in bioengineering research. **Summa Health System**

point, we had no good ways of knowing what was going on in the joint surface of arthritic knees."

The Institute for Biomedical Engineering Research

As a medical school senior at Ohio State, Gradisar had worked with Ernest Johnson on a research project in which he used an oscilloscope to record knee sounds in patients who were to have surgery the following day. After surgery, he recalled, "we'd go back, retrieve the operative reports and any other pertinent laboratory data. We classified these sounds according to the diagnosis discovered in surgery and began to make some sense of that." Back at City after postgraduate work with Dr. Burstein, Gradisar joined forces with Mamerto Chu, Ph.D. of the University of Akron's Mechanical Engineering Department. The two continued "to develop a non-invasive test for assessing articular knee cartilage. We applied for N.I.H. funding and received several hundred thousand dollars to carry on that research. We published a number of papers. About the time the technique became fairly useful, the arthroscope came along. It gave us a minimally invasive mechanism for optically looking at the joint surface, making this more technically driven, acoustical method less valuable. Nevertheless, we learned a lot."

This noninvasive research project had a serendipitous outcome because "it pointed up the need for us to have better access to the University of Akron," Gradisar said. That need led to the establishment of the Institute for Biomedical Engineering Research. "Dr. Chu from Mechanical Engineering, Dr. Mostardi from Biology, and I worked together," Gradisar continued. "As the engineering college increased enrollment, it was tougher to get faculty released to work on research projects. It was a real dilemma; our research started and stopped, started and stopped. There was also the problem of not having a single spokesman. If we were working in mechanical engineering, for instance, and needed a piece of electrical engineering equipment, we couldn't always get it."

Gradisar, Chu, and Mostardi met with the then University Provost,

Coleman Major, Ph.D., Dean of the U. of A.'s College of Engineering, was the Institute's first Director. He was succeeded by Robin E. Herron, Ph.D., who came from Baylor University in Houston in November 1979 to become IBER's first full-time Director. Besides Dr. Major, the founding Institute members include Mamerto L. Chu, Ph.D., U. of A.'s Mechanical Engineering Department; Alan Gent, Ph.D., Institute of Polymer Science; Ivan A. Gradisar, Jr., M.D.; Walter A. Hoyt, Jr., M.D.; Noel Leathers, Ph.D., University of Akron Provost; Robert Liebelt, M.D., Dean of the Northeastern Ohio College of Medicine (NEOUCOM); George Malindzak, Ph.D., Department of Physiology, NEOUCOM; Richard A. Mostardi, Ph.D., U. of A. Department of Biology; Norman Taslitz, M.D., NEOUCOM's Department of Anatomy.

Noel Leathers, who suggested that the three "develop a solution," which they did. "We needed an institute," Gradisar said, "which would allow the University to work in a coordinated fashion on biomedical research. One which would recognize the unique problems in trying to interface a hospital with an engineering department. Dr. Dominic Guzzetta, President of the University, liked the concept. It was advanced by Dr. Liebelt who was then Dean of the Medical School, and Dr. Hoyt, who was Chairman of the Department of Orthopaedics at City. Dr. Robin Herron, from Baylor University was hired [to head the Institute], co-funded by City Hospital and the University. That is how the Institute for Biomedical Research began in 1979."

The IBER has evolved over the years and is today a component of the U. of A.'s Department of Biomedical Engineering. Dr. Gradisar calls it "a valuable asset to the community, a strong academic program that produces bioengineers who are employed in hospitals and industry. It's one of sixty bioengineering programs in the country and it really began as a solution to a problem that existed between researchers here at City Hospital and faculty members at the University of Akron. There's a terrific amount of cooperation among the medical school, the hospitals, and the University," Gradisar concluded.

City's Musculoskeletal Research Laboratory

Following the guidelines written for the newly formed Institute, the orthopaedists established City Hospital's 2,200-square-foot Musculoskeletal Research Laboratory. It was located on the second floor of the Medical Building, next to the Physical Fitness and Testing Center. Richard A. Mostardi, Ph.D., the Musculoskeletal Research Laboratory's first Director, was granted released time from the University of Akron to work with the clinicians.

The laboratory was busy from the beginning. Arne Melby, III, M.D., collaborated with Narander P. Reddy, Ph.D. and Daniel B. Sheffer, Ph.D., of the

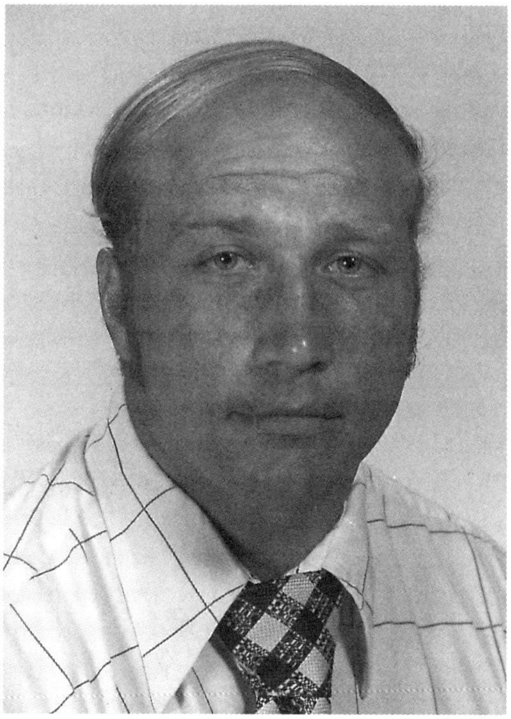

Arne Melby. Through the years, Dr. Melby has been a highly productive researcher and teacher.

Summa Health System

IBER on studies of knee kinematics. Dr. Melby, a fine clinician and teacher, is one of the most productive researchers in orthopaedics at Summa Health System. Drs. Gradisar, Hoyt, Kepley, and Mostardi undertook follow-up studies of hip and knee replacements. In collaboration with William Sharp, M.D. (son of H. Vernon Sharp, M.D., who, with Dr. Steinke, had established City's first animal research laboratory fifty years earlier), Stephen Schmidt, Ph.D., of City's Vascular Research Laboratory, and Bruce Taylor, Ph.D., of City's Medical Engineering Department, began studies in the musculoskeletal laboratory on blood pressure measurement. Daniel Bethem, M.D., began studies of surgical techniques to correct spinal deformities in collaboration with Dr. Mostardi and Michael Savage, Ph.D., of the U. of A.'s Mechanical Engineering Department. Dr. Bethem's paper, "Spinal Deformities of Dwarfism," given at the 16th Scoliosis Research Society Meeting in 1981, is one of the most frequently quoted works on dwarfism as it relates to spinal deformities.

Richard Mostardi joined with James Porterfield, L.P.T., Director of the Physical Fitness and Testing Center, to conduct physical performance evaluations on members of the Ohio Ballet, high school football players, swimmers, and the City of Akron's police and fire fighters. The safety forces typically placed an age restriction on hiring. According to Dr. Gradisar, "Dr. Mostardi did not regard that as an appropriate determination. He set about developing criteria that evaluated the performance level of a person, male or female, old or young, in terms of their ability to carry out the physical responsibilities of a fire fighter or police officer. That's a landmark activity. Dr. Mostardi has testified around the country with his research in regard to people who felt discriminated against because of age. He's also established an intervention program. It evaluates current safety workers whose physical skills may not be up to the level that is recommended for their own safety and their ability to do their work."

City's "On-Board Ph.D."

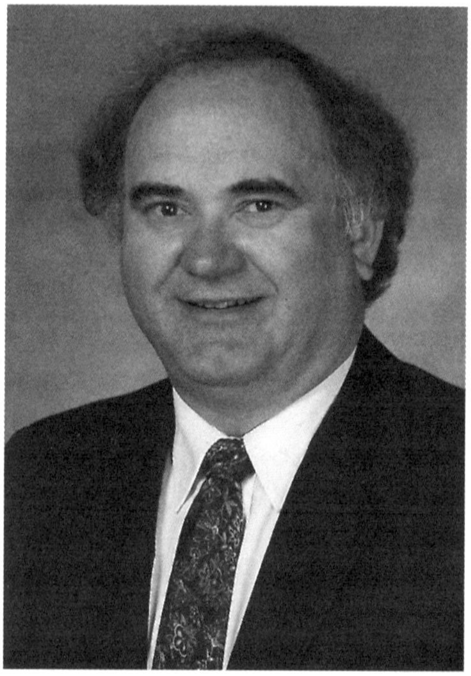

Michael J. Askew. Dr. Askew has directed City Hospital's Musculoskeletal Research Laboratory for fifteen years.
Summa Health System

The three-way collaboration of university, institute, and orthopaedists was successful, but something was missing. Dr. Gradisar's fellowship at Case Western Reserve taught him that "having a bioengineer on site [at the hospital] would enrich the teaching and educational research opportunities in the department. It would be a real asset to an orthopaedic training program." Could they afford it? Did they have the infrastructure to sustain such a program? Was the academic material here? "I suggested to Dr. Hoyt that we take a good, hard look at it," Gradisar said. "We decided that a site review by Dr. Albert Burstein would be a valuable first step."

Dr. Burstein spent several days at City Hospital in 1981, interviewing orthopaedists and people from the University. He looked at the issue very closely and "recommended that City's orthopaedic research residency program did have the capacity to sustain a bioengineering research laboratory and recommended that it be established," Gradisar recalled. "He also agreed to help identify that laboratory's first director. With Dr. Burstein's help, we set up a national search for a Ph.D. to head the laboratory. We were fortunate to find Dr. Michael Askew who agreed to come and really establish the laboratory." On March 1, 1983, Michael J. Askew, Ph.D., of the Rehabilitation Engineering Program at Northwestern University Medical School in Chicago, became the first full-time director of the Musculoskeletal Research Laboratory.

City's renovated Musculoskeletal Research Laboratory opened on April 11, 1983, with Mrs. Margaret Ireland as the secretary. Someone has to pay the bills and many "someones," physicians and lay people, have aided research and education at City Hospital for many years. Contributors include the Calhoun Trust, City Hospital, the Corbin Foundation, the Howland Foundation, the Knight Foundation, the Lowell-Hoyt-Steinke Fund, the Charles and Mabel Ritchie Foundation, the Robertson-Hoyt Fund, the Showalter Trust, Summa Health Foundation, and donations from Ella Iredell, M.G. O'Neil, and E.J. Thomas.

Dr. Gradisar is the only one of his peers to take a fellowship in bio-

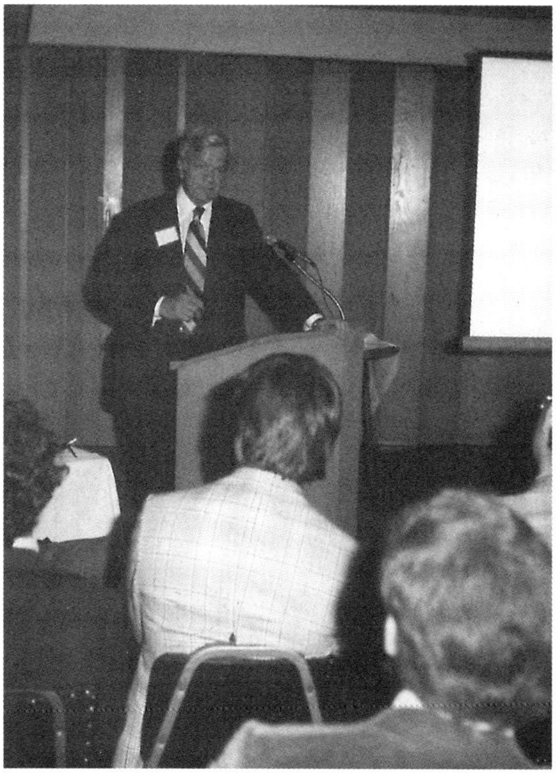
Dr. Hoyt (background) makes a point at a resident conference.
Summa Health System

engineering. As Medical Director of Research in Summa's Department of Orthopaedic Surgery, Gradisar balances a busy practice with a series of research projects. "We have no paid physicians [including himself] involved in any of the research work done in the department," he said. "Our people come to the lab simply because they have the intellectual curiosity to show up and answer a question."

Some would argue that a more conventional medical environment, such as at the University of Chicago or Johns Hopkins, with their university hospitals and tenured faculty, do more sophisticated research. Dr. Gradisar acknowledges that is true. "But," he says, "our research is primarily targeted at the clinical outcome level."

Orthopaedic research at Summa "has a very short loop," Gradisar said. "It is applied research that begins with a clinical question developed by an active practitioner. It goes to the laboratory for better understanding and resolution and the answer comes right back to the patient. A dollar spent here has a very quick, immediate impact on health care delivery in Summit County and northeastern Ohio. This community gets a big bang for its buck; they have a first rate medical environment without paying the freight for faculty. These are private practitioners who see patients, but get involved with research and education purely on a voluntary basis."

Research benefits the residents throughout their professional lives. "You want residents to be critical listeners and critical readers," Gradisar said, "that's the first target. You can't do that until you've been in a laboratory and encountered first hand the difficulty of getting accurate information. The ABOS recommends that strong evidence of scholarly effort in a particular research project be done in a program in order to maintain accreditation. We met that requirement for years simply by conducting research as a standard portion of every day's activity. We published papers for years and years prior to the advent of the laboratory and the Akron City Hospital Foundation. With

Foundation funding, however, with the laboratory space, and the on-board Ph.D., now we could make it part of the residents' rotation."

Win, Win, Win Situations

Patients benefit most of all. Early in the seventies, Dr. Edmund Chao, a bioengineer at the Mayo Clinic, recommended to Dr. Gradisar that he work with manufacturers of the joint implants he uses. Interviewed in 1996, Gradisar explained that "Chao's recommendation allows us to examine patients in a follow-up. Over the years," he continued, "when we've switched to a total knee or total hip of a certain design, we've gone back to the company through Dr. Askew, and recommended that the company fund a follow-up of these patients. So, typically, we bring these private patients back to the Musculoskeletal Research Laboratory two years after surgery. They have X-rays and evaluation by the research lab staff who perform a protocol follow-up evaluation of each patient. The reports are collated and sent back to the company, which now has a scientific evaluation of the performance of their particular product in my patients. Frequently, we write a paper on the outcome. And, the patient has a free follow-up. So, it's a win, win, win situation. Ours is one of the earliest examples of 'outcomes research,' a concept now newly discovered and in vogue around the country. We've been doing it at Summa since the mid-seventies."

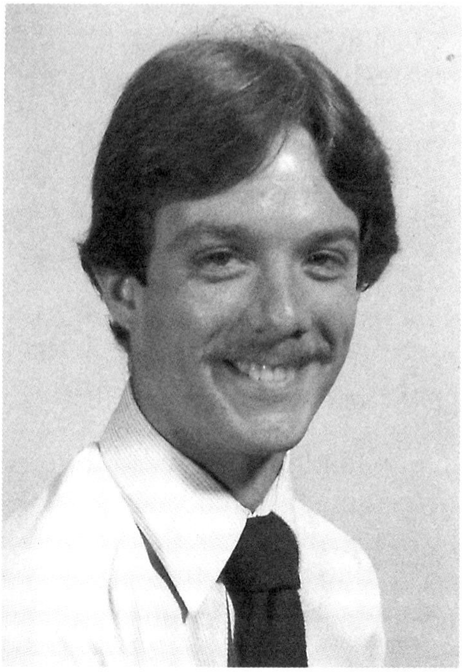

Paul R. Fleissner, Jr. Dr. Fleissner's paper "Mechanical Properties of Antibiotic Impregnated Bone Cement" won awards locally and at the Ohio Orthopaedics Society Annual Meeting in Cleveland. **Summa Health System**

In October 1998, shortly before he departed for Australia to lecture and perform surgery, Dr. Gradisar described another "win, win, win" situation which holds bright prospects for patients. In this instance, he reviewed the collaboration of academicians and clinicians at the University of Akron's Department of Engineering, Summa Health System, and the Northeastern Ohio Universities College of Medicine (NEOUCOM) and demonstrated how, by working together, each benefits the other. "For the Musculoskeletal Research Laboratory, [the collaboration] meant access to basic science technology, specialized laboratory testing equipment, and engineering expertise," Gradisar said. "To the University, it meant projects for undergraduate and graduate students because it gave them an opportunity for collaborative research funding applications that neither institution could acquire if they did not apply for funds jointly. This coordination between the University and the Musculoskeletal Research Laboratory at Summa, under the direction of Dr. Askew, resulted in a number of graduate theses and collaborative research in multiple areas, including acoustical emissions of the knee, the development of new bone cements, the evaluation of energy absorbing polymers as shoe inserts, the development of wrestling mats with special shock absorbing characteristics, etc."

"The collaboration between NEOUCOM researchers and the Musculoskeletal Research Laboratory is more recent," Gradisar continued. "The medical school's vivarium is a very valuable resource and has been used for a long time. But, it wasn't until the last seven to ten years that bona fide interaction in research has occurred. The medical school's addition of basic scientists with expertise in bone and cartilage research has stimulated what promises to be a very strong source of interaction. Significant contributions are expected from the basic science strength at the medical school coupled with the access to pathology and clinical strengths at the hospital. The Musculoskeletal Research Laboratory will likely be the linchpin in that coordination."

In his 1996 interview, Dr. Gradisar said that when he starts a project, he recruits a resident to participate and "a lot of good things happen. The resident learns about research and gets a paper. About 60 percent to 70 percent of our residents go on to fellowship programs and the resident who's published gets a leg up in the sought-after fellowships. Most of my research has been affiliated with a resident, developing a paper on a certain theme."

Paul R. Fleissner, M.D., City, class of '89, is one of those who worked with Dr. Gradisar and produced a paper, "Mechanical Properties of Antibiotic Impregnated Bone Cement." Dr. Fleissner received the 1988 Walter A. Hoyt Award for Basic Science Research and the Cleveland Orthopaedic Award for his work. "We wanted to determine whether or not mixing an antibiotic with PMMA, polymethylmethacrilate bone cement, affected its strength," Gradisar said. "Our research showed it does not weaken the cement, the antibiotic stays active, and it's a safe thing to do. That's what the research was intended to determine."

Since its creation in 1979, City's Musculoskeletal Research Laboratory has published thirty-seven papers in refereed journals, has published in fifty additional publications, and has had its work presented at 105 national, regional, and local presentations. Residents have made thirty-four of these presentations and ten have received awards for their research.

Research is fun on two days, according to Dr. Gradisar. "The day you discover the question and the day you find the answer! In between, it's just a lot of sweat and frustration. But, once in a while, a resident will find that ecstatic moment supportive enough that they'll labor through the frustration to an answer. That's the bird you're looking for in the training program."

Musculoskeletal research has entered a new phase. "The mechanical engineering solutions of the past are not the central area of inquiry now," Gradisar said in his 1996 interview. "Engineering is beginning to take on a very strong biological tint. The cellular elements, the biological aspects of engineering, are center stage. Publications coming out of the laboratory now have a lot to do with cellular debris and the biological response to that. So, we're changing with the times and beginning to ask questions that are occurring to other clinicians around the country, cellular questions."

Changing with the times has been the rule for three generations of Akron's orthopaedists because they understand that the best patient care is founded on a strong educational background and solid research. The Northeastern Ohio Universities College of Medicine provided the base for an academic infrastructure that brought the clinician and the academician together and allowed the residencies to grow and flourish. In the eighties, the second generation passed the torch to the third, many of whom took fellowships, subspecialized, and returned to lead these programs into the 21st century.

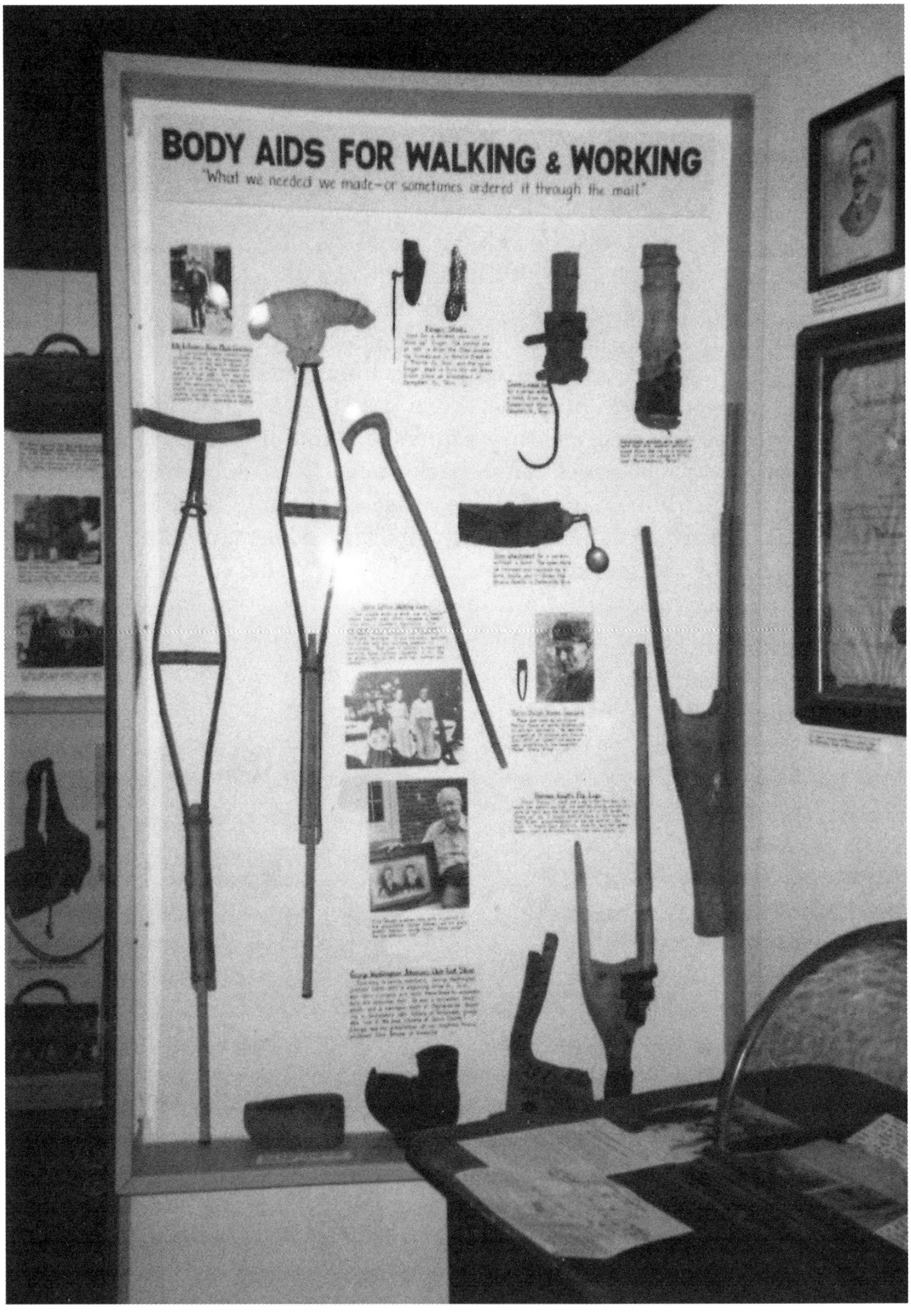

The Museum of Appalachia in Norris, Tennessee. A century ago, prosthetics and orthotics were simply "Body Aids for Walking and Working."
Photo by Marcia Kanis, Akron General Medical Center

Chapter Four

1983-1997, "A New, Exciting Golden Era"

By the 1980's, subspecialization had become the standard both in orthopaedics education and in practice. As had been the case throughout the twentieth century (and especially after the Second World War), scientists around the world were continuing to increase the fund of medical knowledge, creating sophisticated technology that supported a host of new surgical procedures. Simultaneously, new leaders entered the scene in the Rubber City. At Akron General Medical Center, Buel S. Smith succeeded Harry O'Dell in 1975 and served until 1993 when Mark C. Leeson, AGMC, class of '83, succeeded him. Dennis S. Weiner, AGMC, class of '69, succeeded W.A. Hoyt, Jr. in 1980 as Chairman of Children's Hospital Medical Center's Department of Orthopaedics. J. Patrick Flanagan, City, class of '73, succeeded Hoyt as Chairman of City Hospital's Department of Orthopaedics in 1984.

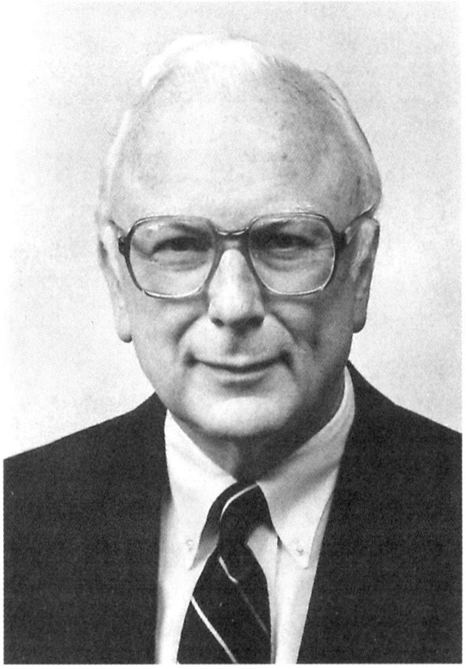

Buel Smith. Dr. Smith served in both orthopaedic residency programs and chaired Akron General Medical Center's Department of Orthopaedics for eighteen years.
Akron General Medical Center

Change came to the Northeastern Ohio Universities College of Medicine, too. Buel Smith succeeded Walter Hoyt as Chairman of the Council of Chiefs of Orthopaedic Surgery at NEOUCOM in 1982 and served until 1993, when he was succeeded by Pat Flanagan. The Orthopaedic Council reached an agreement with the Council of Surgery in 1983 that orthopaedic surgery would be one of the electives available to the third year students during their basic course in surgery. Besides "improving the students' exposure to all aspects of modern surgery," Smith says, "the curriculum change greatly increased the interaction between the students and the orthopaedic faculty."

Akron was the Rubber Capital of the World for the first three quarters of the twentieth century. In the late 1970's, however, one by one, the big rubber companies moved away, leaving thousands jobless. The advent of the radial tire was one factor in the exodus. Also, the Rubber City's antiquated facto-

Dr. Smith served on a number of committees at NEOUCOM over the years. Like his predecessor, Dr. Hoyt, his interests ranged beyond his specialty. He served as a member of the Academic Council, he was a member of the Committee on Committees for two terms as well as the Committee on Continuing Medical Education. Smith chaired the Faculty Appointments and Promotions Committee for six years prior to 1994 and under his leadership, the committee changed and greatly improved procedures for appointments and promotions during this period. At Commencement in 1994, he received the President's Award for service to the College.

ries, a history of labor unrest, and the lure of modern plants in warmer, union-free climes combined to end the old mill town's dominance as a tire producer. The city succeeded in redefining itself in the post-industrial age, emerging in the nineties as a white collar, service oriented metropolis some have nicknamed "Polymer Heights," (recognizing area expertise in polymer science). In 1994, according to George Knepper's book, *Akron, City at the Summit*, "among the top ten employers, companies that make things employ just 11,350 persons; those that provide services employ 24,114."

Two of those top ten employers serving the community are Akron General Medical Center and Summa Health System. St. Thomas Hospital and City Hospital merged in March 1989 to form Summa Health System. City had been planning yet another major building program in 1988 to accommodate its growing patient population. Meanwhile, St. Thomas experienced a drop in its census. The merger consolidated services and, after much discussion, City's Department of Orthopaedics moved to St. Thomas in 1993. The orthopaedic department's offices, musculoskeletal research laboratory, and surgical suites had been scattered throughout different buildings on City's sprawling campus. Now, the department is consolidated in one place. As Dr. Gradisar observed in October 1994 at the dedication of the Walter A. Hoyt, Jr., M.D., Musculoskeletal Laboratory: "For the first time in the history of this institution, the facilities match the skill and competence of the orthopaedic staff, nurses, technicians, therapists, etc."

Dr. Hoyt stepped down as Chairman of Akron City Hospital's Department of Orthopaedic Surgery in 1982. In February of that year, he addressed the new Fellows of the American Academy of Orthopaedic Surgeons. In a talk about change and continuity Hoyt stressed the basics, "four important parts of your life as an orthopaedic surgeon." To illustrate this theme, he chose the homely four-legged-stool that is "mostly unsat upon" in the operating room. EDUCATION, RESEARCH, PATIENT CARE are three legs of the four legged stool. The first leg is EDUCATION, continuing education, that is. "You must educate yourself and apply what you learn to your patients who need you." The second leg, RESEARCH, "has brought orthopaedics to a high level of patient service." The third leg, PATIENT CARE, offers "the opportunity to apply your knowledge and skills acquired over the last twenty-five years. It is the epitome of being a physician." These three legs require the Hard Sciences. "You need your Intelligence Quotient, your I.Q., to take it all in," as the Hard Sciences in the form of new techniques, equipment, procedures come along.

QUALITY, the stool's fourth leg, is "maybe the most important...and certainly the least talked about..." QUALITY concerns the soft sciences. "A Soft Science is something inside of you that never loses sight of the fact that the body you are working on is more than a case, it's a human being. You need your Q.Q., your Quality Quotient, to succeed in the Soft Sciences. We all know some of these Soft Science Words...encouragement, awareness of others, sympathy, compassion...not just care of the patient, but caring for the patient."

Hoyt's second theme in "The Four Legged Stool" concerns the forward-looking attitude that has sustained Akron's programs through the years and helped them deal with medicine's myriad changes. Here, he recognized the "restrictions of third party payers, regulations imposed by Government and others, the problems of hospital finance, and insurance," and put them in perspective: "In my past, I've had freedom to function according to my own conscience. That was good. But I also worked in an era when surgical instruments, by today's standards, might be called primitive. So, times have changed."

While regretting "the decline of autonomous medical practices of a few decades ago, I accept these truths: Today's operating rooms and techniques have dramatically improved. Surgical instruments answer our needs better than ever before...our knowledge base has expanded beyond the capability of any one individual's ability to assimilate...and best of all: our patients have a better prognosis. We are making people better. Could we ask for anything beyond that?"

For Dr. Hoyt, there was no looking back, "wanting the good old days...the Golden Era of the past. I like it," he told Academy members, "that there is now more information, more quickly shared by computer, by fax, and by phone. I like it that we can electronically consult with physicians around the world. I like it that in our x-ray reading rooms we can study computer graphics and readouts, surely going more below the surface than we were ever able to do before. Yes. I like it that we know there are good things ahead and that this is just the beginning of a new, exciting Golden Era emerging."

Assembling a Faculty in the 1980's and 1990's

The desire to become more proficient in caring for patients is part of medicine's armamentarium and fellowship training is simply another step in

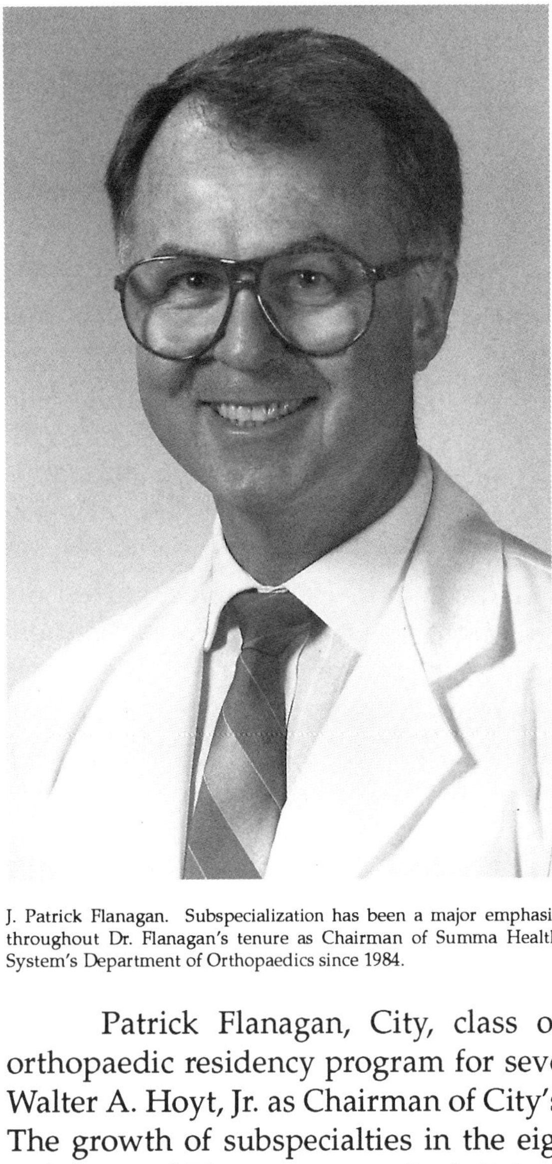

J. Patrick Flanagan. Subspecialization has been a major emphasis throughout Dr. Flanagan's tenure as Chairman of Summa Health System's Department of Orthopaedics since 1984.

sharpening skills. Over the last century, each era in the development of orthopaedic surgery has begun with a preceptorship. In the teens, twenties, and thirties, general surgeons studied orthopaedics under an accomplished bone and joint surgeon; in the sixties and seventies, general orthopaedists apprenticed themselves to subspecialists; and, by the 1980's, postgraduate training had evolved from physicians designing their own fellowships to accredited programs listed by the American Academy of Orthopaedic Surgeons in an inch-thick book. Having built their academic base in the 1970's, Akron's orthopaedists assembled a faculty strong in subspecialists who became the linchpin of both programs. Today, as Donald Beringer, M.D., Summa, class of '96, said, "the heart and soul of the residency program is in the strength of the subspecialists."

Patrick Flanagan, City, class of '73, had directed City Hospital's orthopaedic residency program for seven years when, in 1984, he succeeded Walter A. Hoyt, Jr. as Chairman of City's Department of Orthopaedic Surgery. The growth of subspecialties in the eighties substantially affected residency training and Flanagan notes "a definite improvement in the residents' conferences because they have moved from residents teaching residents to subspecialists teaching the residents."

While Flanagan concentrated on orthopaedic education, his colleague, Ivan Gradisar, class of '72, helped establish City's orthopaedic research program and, according to Flanagan, "continues to be its driving force. His inquisitive mind and creative thought processes made him an ideal candidate to shepherd the research activities of the Department of Orthopaedics."

In 1983, the Advisory Council for Orthopaedic Resident Education [ACORE], reviewed Akron's programs. Both passed. The reviewer, Dr. John Gartland of Jefferson Medical College, strongly recommended that Akron

General Medical Center develop new subspecialty capabilities. And that is what they did. According to Mark C. Leeson, chairman of AGMC's Department of Orthopaedics, "we developed a hospital-based group comprised mainly of subspecialists who basically perform the duties of an academic department." (Summa's program is organized differently; Flanagan, the Chairman, and Scott Weiner, City, class of '91, Director of Education and subspecialist in orthopaedic oncology, are the only hospital-based faculty. The rest are community practitioners, many of whom are subspecialists.) General's new subspecialist base played a role in their program's growth in 1988. They requested a review by the Residency Review Committee and proposed expanding their program from two to three residents per year, beginning at the first year level and reaching a full compliment of fifteen residents in 1995. They understood, according to Buel Smith, then chairman of the department, "that it was extremely difficult to win approval for the expansion of a residency. We were not at all optimistic and were delighted when the Residency Review Committee agreed to this expansion with no additional requirements or questions."

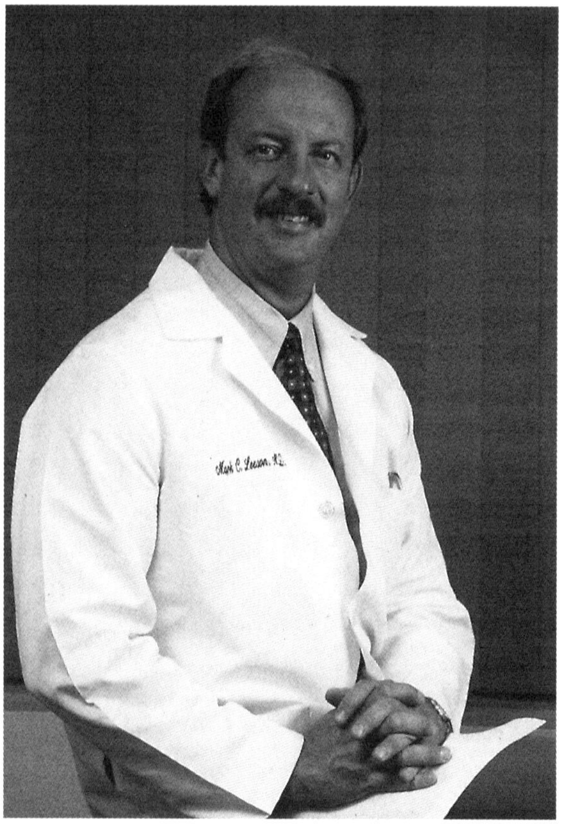

Mark C. Leeson. A dedicated clinician and researcher, Dr. Leeson has presented papers around the world. He serves as Chairman of the Orthopaedic Department of Akron General Medical Center.

In an interview on March 6, 1996, Mark Leeson said that many of Akron General Medical Center's orthopaedic faculty are graduates of that program. They are "handpicked from specific fellowships from all across the country, from Philadelphia in spine and sports medicine to foot and ankle in Dallas, to shoulder in Seattle." James P. Kennedy, AGMC, class of '89, was the first to have a fellowship in major orthopaedic trauma. Gregory Vrabec AGMC, class of '89, recently joined Akron General's orthopaedic department following fellowships in major trauma and total joint replacement. Paul R. Reiman, AGMC, class of '84, followed his residency with a fellowship in arthroscopy and sports medicine, as did John Pinkowski, AGMC, class of '90. David B. Kay, AGMC,

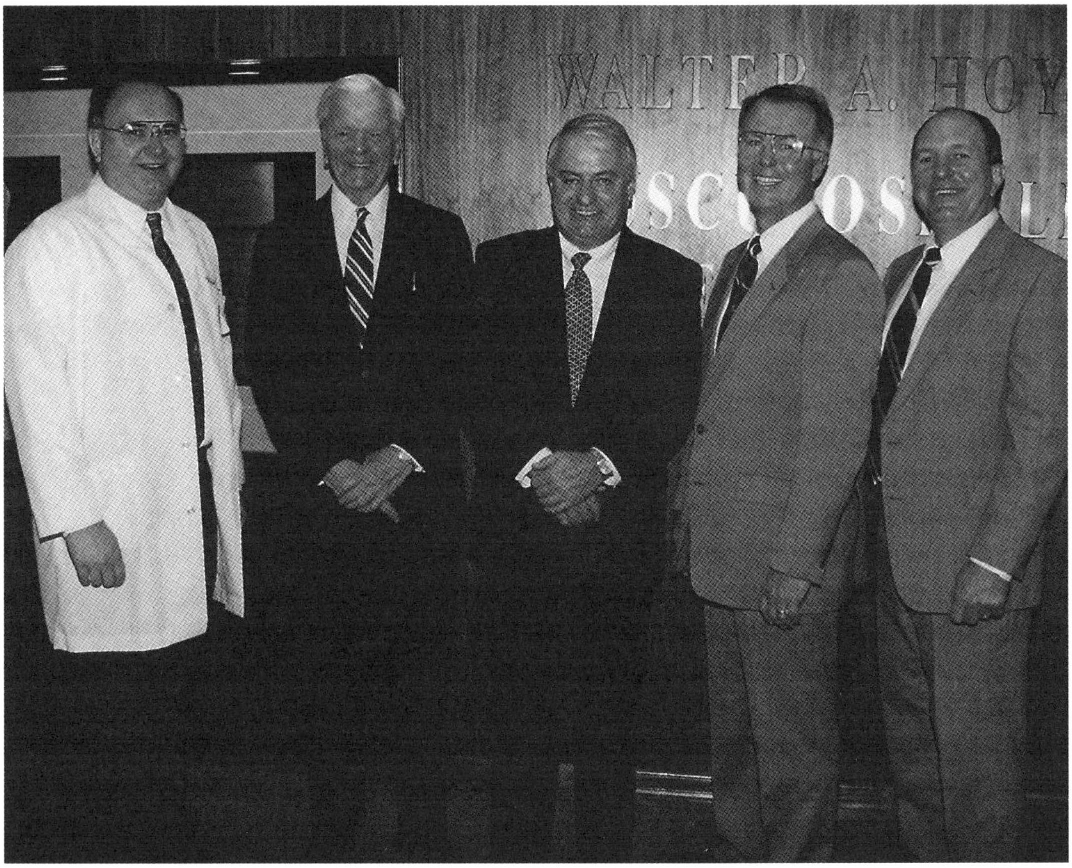

Dedicating the Walter A. Hoyt, Jr., M.D. Musculoskeletal Research Laboratory in October 1994. Left to right: Michael J. Askew, Ph.D., Director of the Laboratory; Walter A. Hoyt, Jr., M.D.; Albert Gilbert, Ph.D., President and C.E.O. of Summa Health System; J. Patrick Flanagan, M.D., Chairman of Summa's Department of Orthopaedics; Ivan A. Gradisar, Jr., M.D., Medical Director of Research at Summa's Department of Orthopaedics. **Summa Health System**

class of '86, completed a fellowship in foot and ankle, and introduced the Ilizarov procedure. Also, Gordon L. Bennett, AGMC, class of '88, took a foot and ankle fellowship. Michael J. Smith, AGMC, class of '91, joined the department after a fellowship in the same subspecialty. Steven B. Lippitt, AGMC, class of '90, completed two years of fellowship at the University of Washington, the first year in shoulder surgery, the second in the administration of an orthopaedic research program. On his return, he became director of General's laboratory. According to Leeson, the University of Washington is "probably the pre-eminent shoulder fellowship in the country. Lippitt is the co-author of two books and is the medical illustrator of those books." The general orthopaedist has not disappeared, however. Thomas Thompson, Michael L. Pryce, AGMC, class of '82, Paul Steurer, and Phillip G. Wilcox, AGMC, class of '85, primarily do general orthopaedics, according to Buel Smith. Michael Pryce took a fellowship in hand and Phillip Wilcox took a fellowship in sports medicine.

Mark Leeson's subspecialty (orthopaedic oncology) exemplifies the encouraging progress achieved over the last twenty years thanks to research and improved technology. Until the mid-seventies, when Leeson was a medical student, almost every patient with a primary tumor of bone or soft tissue received an amputation, whereas reconstruction is the goal today. Leeson took his fellowship in tumors, musculoskeletal oncology, and pathology at Case Western Reserve University and was the first orthopaedic oncologist in Akron. He says that "up until the late seventies, there were no special studies to be able to look at a tumor, look at the size of it, what it was related to, where it was in the muscle, or near nerves or vessels." Technological advances, such as the CAT scan (developed in the late seventies) and the MRI scan (developed in the mid-eighties) "have really helped," Leeson continued, "in making earlier diagnoses. The earlier the diagnosis is, it can support you anatomically in what you can or can't do in terms of removing a tumor and then in terms of what you can or can't do in terms of reconstruction. This interest and increase in technology in terms of earlier diagnosis, better medical management, goes along with better anesthesia, being able to put people to sleep for three, four, six, eight hours at a time and have them not suffer any significant complications. And, there is the team approach, people from internal medicine, radiology, social service, psychology, orthopaedics, working together. All these aspects," Leeson concluded, "play a role in treating not only the disease, but patients and their families."

Akron General Medical Center's orthopaedic research program continues to develop and, according to Dr. Leeson, most of General's orthopaedists have adjunct associate professorships in the U. of A.'s biomedical engineering research department. "We have access to that institution and that research and the personnel, as well as that of the medical school and our own research lab," he said. "We have Dr. Njus, who is a Ph.D. in biomedical engineering who interfaces with us, I suspect, very much as Dr. Askew does at Summa."

Basic science research in orthopaedics continues to flow out of Akron General Medical Center's recently expanded Calhoun Laboratory under the direction of Glen Njus, Ph.D. in biomedical engineering. An energetic, productive researcher, Dr. Njus spent eight years as a biomedical engineer in the Orthopaedic Research Laboratory at the University of Iowa. Buel Smith says that Dr. Njus, besides working on his own projects, "assists the residents in the design of almost any research project." According to Mark Leeson, "the number of projects performed and presented each year nationally, regionally, and locally, is phenomenal for a program of this size."

Dr. Leeson is especially pleased that "the residents have such a huge involvement in the research. It's important that they understand what a research project is; how it can be constructed, whether it's prospective, retrospective, blind, a double blind, at random. It's necessary that they do research. When they are in practice, faced with reading and reviewing several hundred pages of journal material each month, they'll be able to assimilate what's important from those [research] projects into their own practice and their own patient care. It's this involvement with research that you hope they will be able to use over the next thirty years of their practice to make good clinical decisions in regard to their patients. That's where you can really make a difference."

Clinicians and academicians have collaborated over the years to achieve orthopaedics' prime goal: restoring normal function. Akron's orthopaedic oncologists are active members of several "multi-institutional groups," such as the Children's Cancer Study Group and the Eastern Oncologic Group that facilitate this collaboration. "Obviously, the goal in tumor management," Leeson said, "is to obtain the best prognosis, the best survival. To do that, we're always looking for newer and new, better ways to manage patients with chemotherapy protocols, surgery protocols, how to put those two together. If you have everybody in the country doing one or two cases in a certain way, it's difficult to collect statistically significant data and then make any clear determination of what good ways there are to improve care. All you really have then is a lot of isolated individuals who are doing things, quote, unquote, 'their way,' which may or may not be good or reproducible. What the multi-institutional groups allow us to do is enter patients in a combined fashion, to develop protocols through meetings and interactions, to treat a certain group of patients with a certain diagnosis in a specific way for a specific length of time. Then we can determine the results of that treatment in comparison to the results of other treatments, so that you can then make advances in improving care. Until you put science to it, it's all very anecdotal and non-reproducible."

Fellowships offer a one-year period of advanced study at a single institution. A more advanced version, the "travelling fellowship," allows the clinician, as Mark Leeson says, "to spend short periods of time at several institutions in the arena of their subspecialty." Leeson received a travelling fellowship grant from the Mid-America Orthopaedic Association and says "the ideal is to take someone who's been doing clinical work and research for four or five years, at least, so that they have patients of their own and have seen where their problems lie. It's really exploring around the country at three or four places, seeing what those institutions are doing, how they manage those particular sets of problems, or to share the information that you perhaps have developed with them. It's a little more personal than at a meeting in which there are three hundred people attending."

The attendings benefit from participating in the programs as much as the residents. Community orthopaedists, such as Tom Bear, find that Summa's program is a two-way street on which the teacher is also the student. Bear credits the residency program with helping him "stay abreast, or ahead of, what the residents are studying and learning. If you're going to practice with them and teach them, you have to keep up and stay ahead. A number of residents have stimulated me to branch out or advance my technique and knowledge. When I look at knee surgery, I can start with Bill Heyerman, Bill Mahon, Tim Meyer, Bruce Holladay, and Chris Klonk. Joint replacement, I think of residents in their senior year who stimulated me to move ahead. Bob Kepley, who's now my partner, and Joe Berman."

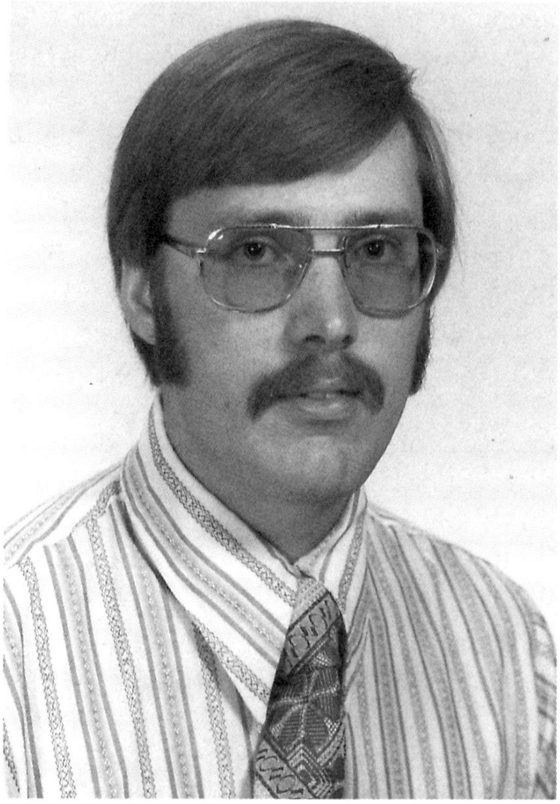

Robert F. Kepley. Dr. Kepley took his fellowship in total joint replacement under Dr. Thomas Mallory in Columbus, Ohio.
Summa Health System

"These people pushed the envelope," Bear said, "tried to see where things were going. They encouraged me to go out and advance my technique by scrubbing with pioneers. Townley, Capelo, Hungerford, Charles Eng, Larry Dorr, Aaron Hoffman, Tom Mallory in Columbus, are people I've scrubbed with, pioneers in the field, to improve my technique. Pat Flanagan is a stimulator. It's been very challenging to remain a member of the teaching staff in his training program. These are things that have drawn me into the community, made me active in the community, made me stay in the community, and made me glad I practiced here rather than someplace else."

Subspecialization occurs in community practices, too. During his residency, Robert Kepley, M.D., City, class of '80, became interested in total joint replacement working with W.A. Hoyt, Jr. and Bill Davis. "There were only two or three established joint replacement fellowships then," Kepley said, "and Dr. Tom Mallory in Columbus had one of them. I did my fellowship with him before starting my practice with Summit Orthopaedic Group, which included Drs. George Mallo, Herb Thompson, and Jim Roberts."

Kepley now practices with Tom Bear. Most of his practice is total joints, "but I still do arthroscopic surgery, foot and ankle, trauma. All of us, when we start out, do everything we were trained to do. But, as we become busier, we become more selective, eliminating what we may not be comfortable with, or what we may not enjoy. We all try to be very appropriate to what's best for the patient; we follow that to the letter of the law here in Akron. And, in great measure, that's why we've subspecialized so much. We're all good at one little thing and we're willing to let the person who's best at it, do it."

Research has developed better instrumentation, better techniques for installing implants, with the result that younger, more active patients are having reconstructive surgery today. "We've improved the actual product of the joint replacement, be it a hip or a knee, to the point that we have more confidence that it will last fifteen or twenty years of that patient's life expectancy," Dr. Kepley said. "Secondly, we have improved our ability to revise a broken, or loose, or worn-out joint and do it successfully and safely. If we get a very young patient that's crippled and in a wheel chair, ten or fifteen years ago we might have said, 'stay in your wheel chair until you're sixty or sixty-five and then we'll fix you. Now we tend to say, get it fixed; this is the prime of your life. We might as well take advantage of it and when it fails, we'll fix it again because we know how to do that."

Subspecialization blossomed in the eighties. Robert H. Bell, M.D., City, class of '84, "wanted to have a private practice and, at the same time, be able to conduct research and work with residents." He interviewed locally, "back home in Milwaukee, a place in Chicago, and one in San Diego. It was really just in this community that I could do all those things." Bell joined Orthopaedic Surgeons, Inc. (now the Crystal Clinic) "with the caveat that I pursue some subspecialty training. They said, 'we want somebody who's subspecialty trained and can bring something back to the community.'"

Bell chose shoulder as his subspecialty, "but there were only three people in the world with whom you could do a shoulder fellowship. One, Rich Hawkins, was up in London, Ontario. Whit Ewing, one of my partners, made a call to Rich and, as luck would have it, his Fellow, who was to start in July '84, had cancelled. So, an opening developed. I called and sight unseen, no curriculum vitae, no record in hand, by virtue of Whit standing up for me, saying 'he's a good guy, will you take him?' Rich Hawkins said yes." Bell moved his family to Ontario for six months and thereafter, in January '85, returned to Akron to go into practice.

At first, some attendings questioned Bell's choice of subspecialty, but when he returned from Ontario, he found himself "doing more shoulder in a month than I saw in my five years as a resident...Today [July 8, 1996] I did a total shoulder replacement. I never heard of one being done here prior to my returning to town. Now, another young orthopaedist in my group, Jeff Noble, is doing shoulder and Steve Lippit, over at Akron General, is trained in shoulder. So, it's become a very popular subspecialty."

The Rubber City's orthopaedists have always shared information with their peers and they have educated themselves where necessary with help and support from their colleagues. Today, this once "forgotten joint," (the shoulder) and a procedure (arthroscopy) that was virtually unknown in North America thirty years ago, have combined to slowly overtake Bell's practice, of which approximately 50 percent is arthroscopic shoulder work. Indeed, arthroscopic surgical procedures make up the majority of elective orthopaedic procedures at Summa, according to Dr. Whit Ewing.

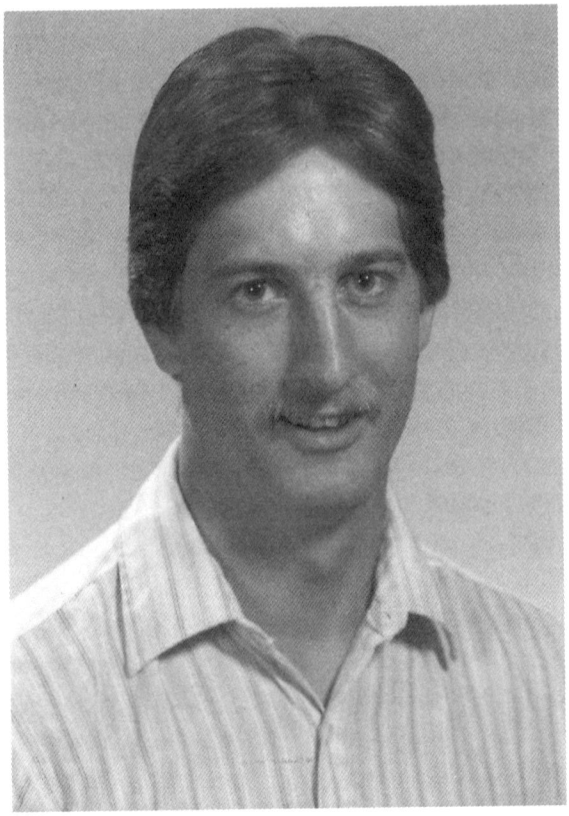

Kenneth A. Greene. Dr. Greene, photographed as an intern, is now Section Chief of Adult Reconstructive Surgery at Summa Health System. **Summa Health System**

Ewing was "on the cusp of the arthroscopic revolution in the early 1980's," Bell says, "performing up to 30 diagnostic knee arthroscopies a week." Developed in Japan in 1918 by Professor Kenji Takagi, advanced by his student, Dr. Masaki Watanabe, in the fifties, arthroscopy was "re-introduced in North America by a Canadian, Dr. Robert Jackson," according to Dr. Ewing.

Kenneth A. Greene, M.D., City, class of '87, took his fellowship at the Cleveland Clinic under the direction of Lester S. Borden, M.D. He also worked with Alan Wilde, M.D., and Bernard N. Stulberg, M.D., but mostly with Dr. Borden. His fellowship was "directed basically at complex and revision total hip and total knee procedures." During his residency, Greene had observed "the huge volume of total joints and total knee replacements coming out of our group, with Gradisar focused on the knee and Hoyt focused on the hip," and spotted a niche doing revision surgery. It was a good choice. "When I came back, touting myself as a revision surgeon, it was amazing the number of cases that were referred to me. Even orthopaedic surgeons we competed with from a business standpoint said, 'well, that's great.' So, though I also do primary hip and knee replacements, I've wound up doing a lot of redo work."

Dr. Greene heads Adult Reconstructive Surgery at Summa. "When the residents rotate on the total joint service, I'm responsible for their education. I lecture at Summa for their residents, I lecture at Akron General for their residency program, and I'm involved with the medical students. You can't quit learning. We give educational seminars for orthopaedic surgeons. We had a total hip meeting [in September 1996] that focused on a new implant. (Greene was one of twenty-five orthopaedists across the country chosen to be an early investigator on this implant.) "We brought people up to speed on that system and allowed them to practice this surgery on prepared dried bones. Education never stops."

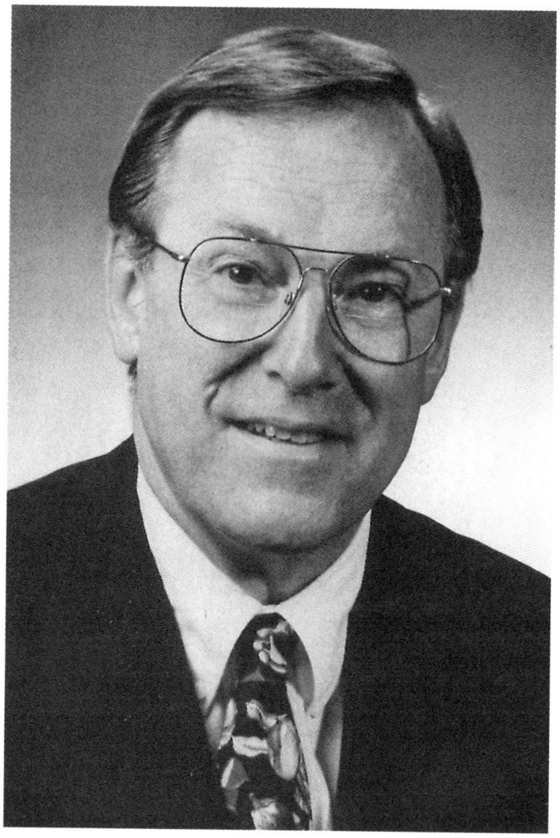

John A. McCulloch. Dr. McCulloch graduated from the University of Toronto (Canada) School of Medicine in June 1963 and has written extensively on spinal surgery.

John A. McCulloch

Greene emphasizes the need for close follow-up on total hip or knee replacement patients to be sure that the implant's plastic liner is not wearing away. If caught in time, it is a thirty minute operation to replace the worn liner in the knee versus a two and a half hour surgery to replace the implant. "Even if the patient doesn't hurt," he said, "it's still important to follow them with an X-ray because they may start wearing the plastic out and not have any pain." Some patients need a bit closer following than others. One of Greene's patients, a man in his seventies, competes in the race walks in the National Senior Olympics, "which isn't too traumatic on a total hip replacement," Greene said. "But, he's also high jumping - on a hip replacement surgery. We ask him to come in at least once a year, have an X-ray, to be sure he's not in trouble."

Not all the faculty are alumni of Akron's orthopaedic residencies. Both programs have always welcomed talented practitioners who bring a fresh perspective to orthopaedic education. Two Canadians, Ian J. Alexander, M.D., foot and ankle subspecialist, and John A. McCulloch, M.D., spine surgery subspecialist, have practiced in Akron since 1990 and 1983, respectively. Each has written extensively on his subspecialty and lectured around the world. Dr. Alexander recently returned from "the medical circuit," as he terms it, lecturing in Australia, sponsored by the Australian Foot and Ankle Society.

Dennis Weiner recalls that "John McCulloch's entry into this community in 1983 added another perspective in an arena where we were just beginning to emerge - the field of spinal surgery. He was one of the pioneers in the use of chymopapain [a proteolytic enzyme used medically in chemonucleolysis - treating a slipped disc with chymopapain to dissolve the displaced nucleus pulposus]. And, he is clearly a pioneer in microsurgery as far as back surgery is concerned."

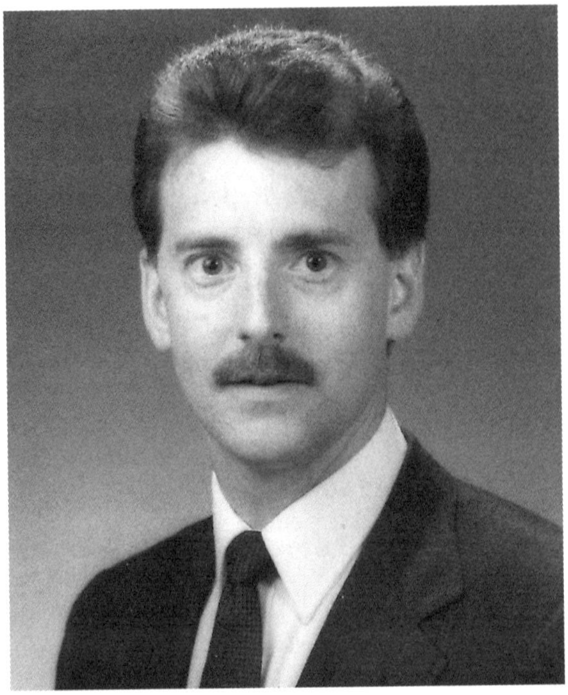

Ian J. Alexander. Dr. Alexander graduated from University of Western Ontario's School of Medicine in 1978 and specializes in foot and ankle surgery.

Doctors McCulloch and Alexander are the only physicians to have directed a fellowship each in Akron. As a rule, the local orthopaedic attendings do not offer postgraduate work (fellowships), preferring to concentrate on their strong graduate programs. For example, Dennis Weiner, a pediatric orthopaedist, "has stayed away from fellowships, because we want to protect the high quality of our residencies. A Fellow can take time you should be spending with residents [especially in surgery where there are only so many places at the operating table] and the residency sort of loses its edge. We think our best role is to provide the highest level of pediatric orthopaedic training for residents. Then they go away to take their fellowships."

Akron's orthopaedic residency graduates practice throughout the country, and they often return to share knowledge. For instance, Gerald Lang, M.D., Summa, class of '93, took a fellowship in trauma under James F. Kellam, M.D. at the Carolinas Health Center in Charlotte, North Carolina. Now at the University of Wisconsin, Dr. Lang lectured on pelvic ring fractures and led a colloquium on trauma at St. Thomas Hospital in October, 1997.

Mentors

Several generations of physicians have had a hand in educating their successors, and not just in the operating room or lecture hall. Akron's orthopaedic residency programs at Akron General, Children's, and Summa are marked by a generosity of spirit, a collegiality on the part of the attendings, and a willingness to share knowledge. Tom Bear recalls that he, "Bob Patti, and Pat Flanagan hung out our shingles and went into debt in order to practice independently, plus remain on staff at City and Children's, and be very active in the residency program. There had to be a source of patients and there had to be cooperation by the attending staff to allow us to do that."

"Certain people made it very easy for us," Bear continued. "Bill Davis was very supportive of our practice; he sent patients our way. He encouraged his referring physicians to help us out. Jim Parks turned over large chunks of his practice to us. He gave up a lot of calls, he gave up almost all of his trauma to us. Others who helped us at that time included Buel Smith, who became chairman at General. Buel was very supportive of our practice. Walter Brown and George Bischoff, who were getting towards the end of their careers, transferred many of their trauma cases, especially those that came in the middle of the night. Al Buergler, George Mallo, Tom Reef, Bob Clark, and Jim Roberts also helped us build our practice."

Then there is the matter of being accepted by one's peers in the community. "The first year I was in practice," Bear recalled, "a gentleman came to me and I made the diagnosis of a herniated disk. I worked him up, treated him non-operatively with physical therapy, and finally admitted him to the hospital. I had him in traction, we used a lot of traction in those days. In spite of all my efforts, his condition deteriorated. His leg pain got worse, his neurologic deficit increased. I took him to radiology and personally did his myelogram, which showed a large disk. So, I sat down with him and said this is where we are today and you need an operation. And he said to me, 'well, that's fine. I want Dr. Hoyt to do it.' That's not a problem. I'll put in a consult with Dr. Hoyt, which I did."

The resident accompanying Hoyt on the consult the following day told Bear what transpired. "Dr. Hoyt came in, reviewed the chart, did a physical examination on the man, said, 'it's got a problem and you certainly do need a laminectomy and I'll be glad to do it.' And the man said, 'when can you do it?' Hoyt pulled out his book, looked at it, and said, 'well, it looks to me like the first available slot would be in six weeks. Of course,' Dr. Hoyt continued, 'you know you're in the hands of a very competent surgeon and I expect he could probably get to you this week.' The man thanked him, Hoyt left. The man asked me to do his surgery and he did just fine."

According to Dr. Bear, "this kind of behavior among attending staff is extremely unusual, it's very unique to this community. I talk to my residents, who go all over the country, and the atmosphere elsewhere is very competitive. This was Hoyt's way of accepting me as a colleague and supporting me as a colleague. 'Cause he could have put that man on and done him that week, just as easily as I did. And there's no way that kind of behavior takes place in very many communities in this country. But it still goes on here. Sure, we all try to be the best. We're all after our share of the market in this town, but we're all colleagues. You go back to Fowler B. Roberts, Hoyt, Sr. and Jr., Harry O'Dell, Buel Smith, Don Minnig. Those people built the foundation for what we have now. It's an atmosphere I would not want to see change."

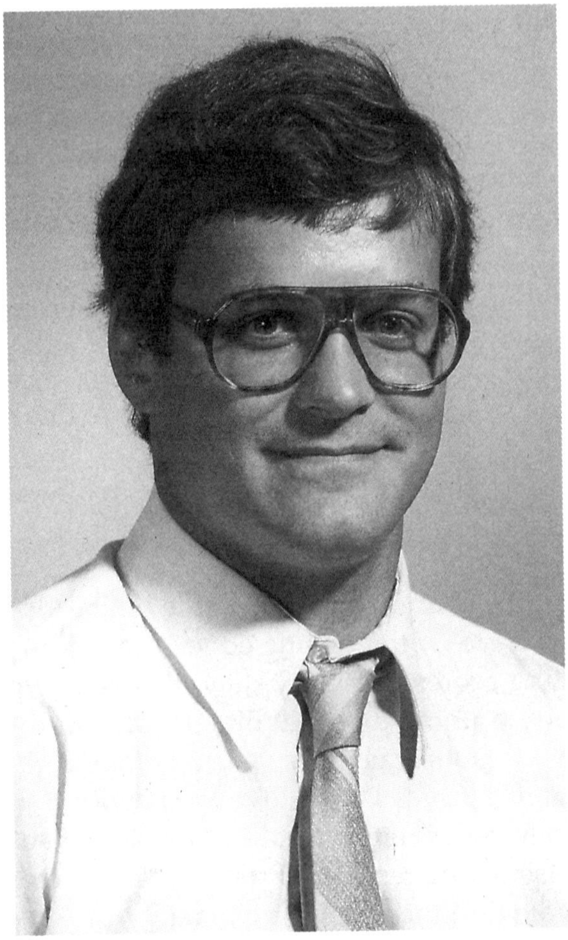

Scott D. Weiner. Dr. Weiner subspecializes in orthopaedic oncology and directs resident education at Summa's Department of Orthopaedics. **Summa Health System**

Though Akron's two orthopaedic residency programs are administered separately, they regularly combine in a very important way: to share knowledge. Mark Leeson says that he and "Dr. Flanagan co-operate to the nth degree. For example, we have a basic science curriculum that we share. We write the curriculum, we review it, change it every two years, add to it, subtract from it. It's at Children's, Wednesdays, from seven in the morning to eight-thirty and residents from all programs go. We share the pediatric exposure and curriculum. We share the hand surgery service curriculum. We share our Visiting Professors. We don't schedule them on top of each other; we try to coordinate them. Both programs are invited so that we get the maximum benefit. This [1997] is the eleventh year that we've had a combined Research Day. All the residents present research they're doing, the projects they're working on, and the clinical and basic science faculty from both institutions review and critique them." Research Day ends on a relaxing note, with golf and dinner.

According to Pat Flanagan, "development of the Akron Orthopaedic Research Day is directly related to the influence of Dennis Weiner. The first combined Akron City, Akron General meeting occurred in 1986 at Children's Hospital. The importance of research in residency education was best expressed by Dr. Weiner in his introductory address to the first resident research meeting: 'What separates a good quality residency training program from a great residency is the ability to conduct and publish quality research that is scrutinized by ones' peers. The programs in Akron have the capacity to achieve such greatness.'"

Self-described "fan" of this community's orthopaedic residency programs, Dennis Weiner took his residency at Akron General Hospital and Akron Children's. According to Dr. Weiner, the residency programs "at both Akron City and Akron General, combined with Akron Children's, have produced residents that are at the highest level of achievement in the United States. In addition, all residents are involved in research projects, and it's mandated. We have a community with excellent patient care, combined with a high level of academic achievement, with research going on on a day to day basis. Add all this up and you have one of the best training programs in all of North America."

Indeed, Dr. Weiner jokes that he would like to have the opportunity to train here "as it is now. And I did train here like it was then. And it wasn't bad then; it's just that it's so much better now. Every single subspecialty is covered in this community now at the highest level it can be by orthopaedic surgeons who are on the cutting edge of their specialty. Many who've come here as visiting professors really stand in awe of what's been accomplished in a community training program like Summa and Akron General."

One can only speculate about what the founding generation, physicians such as W.A. Hoyt, Sr., Fowler B. Roberts, and A.E. Davis, would say if they could return to today's world of subspecialization, high technology, and fascinating research. Probably, they would be interested in it all and pleased to note that the spirit of collegiality they fostered still prevails. And, one likes to think they would be proud of what their successors have built.

It is Match Day, mid-March 1996. Medical school seniors gather in auditoriums nationwide to learn where they will take their residencies. They applied to programs last September and travelled to interviews in November. Now they nervously await the envelope whose contents sets the course of their professional lives.

Others also wait on Match Day. Among them, Mark C. Leeson, M.D. and J. Patrick Flanagan, M.D., Chairmen of the Departments of Orthopaedic Surgery at Akron General Medical Center and Summa Health System, respectively. Seven hundred medical school seniors applied for six available slots in Akron's programs in 1996. Leeson and Flanagan interviewed more than one hundred of these applicants and completed lists of their choices six weeks ago, being especially careful with the first ten to fifteen names. Another program, after all, may be the first choice of your first choice. In most instances, though, Akron's programs get their first choices.

Akron General's and Summa's are strong, nationally known programs, as the quality of their residents attests; they are recruited from the top one-fourth of medical school classes. Kenneth Greene, head of adult reconstructive surgery at Summa, teaches the residents and says it "takes a lot of work, a lot of reading, staying one step ahead of these sharp whippersnappers."

Fifteen years have passed since W.A. Hoyt, Jr. gave his speech to the new Fellows of the AAOS and medicine has experienced many, many more changes: a host of sparkling technological developments have come on the scene, accompanied by an alphabet soup of health maintenance organizations, countless debates over medicare and medicaid, and the continuing rise of medical inflation.

Amidst all this change, there is continuity. Reminiscing recently about City's orthopaedic residency program in the early 1960's, Dr. Hoyt recalled the landscape of his old office desk. Stacks of papers, reports, and charts ranged along its surface. On Hoyt's right, he said, "I had a pile of papers here. That was the training program and that was it! We didn't have anything."

Today, supported by NEOUCOM and the University of Akron with its Department of Bioengineering and Institute for Bioengineering Research, Akron's orthopaedic residency programs have many of the characteristics of a major medical center, albeit one not confined to a single campus. Instead, this non-traditional medical center spreads out over miles in northeastern Ohio and within its confines, as around the world, surgical procedures and techniques have dramatically improved over the years and its practitioners have received national recognition for excellence. The July 27, 1998 issue of *US News and World Report*, which featured "America's Best Hospitals," ranked Summa Health System's Department of Orthopaedics 31st on its list of orthopaedic departments nationwide.

Perhaps one's finest legacy is to be succeeded by exceptionally talented people. Previous generations surely achieved their goal of persuading promising young orthopaedists to remain in the Rubber City, help build the departments, and the residencies. As Ivan Gradisar says, "we trained our people, they went out, got fellowships, came back and trained the rest of us." Gradisar's remark illustrates that British term "dintism," which means, 'by sheer dint of doing it,' that cellist Lynn Harrell considers the key to staying ahead of the game in the music world. When Akron's residencies were "...a pile of papers," the doctors kept on going, doing their work, as Harrell said, "with good will and effort day after day, year after year." The results are quality programs and superior medical care.

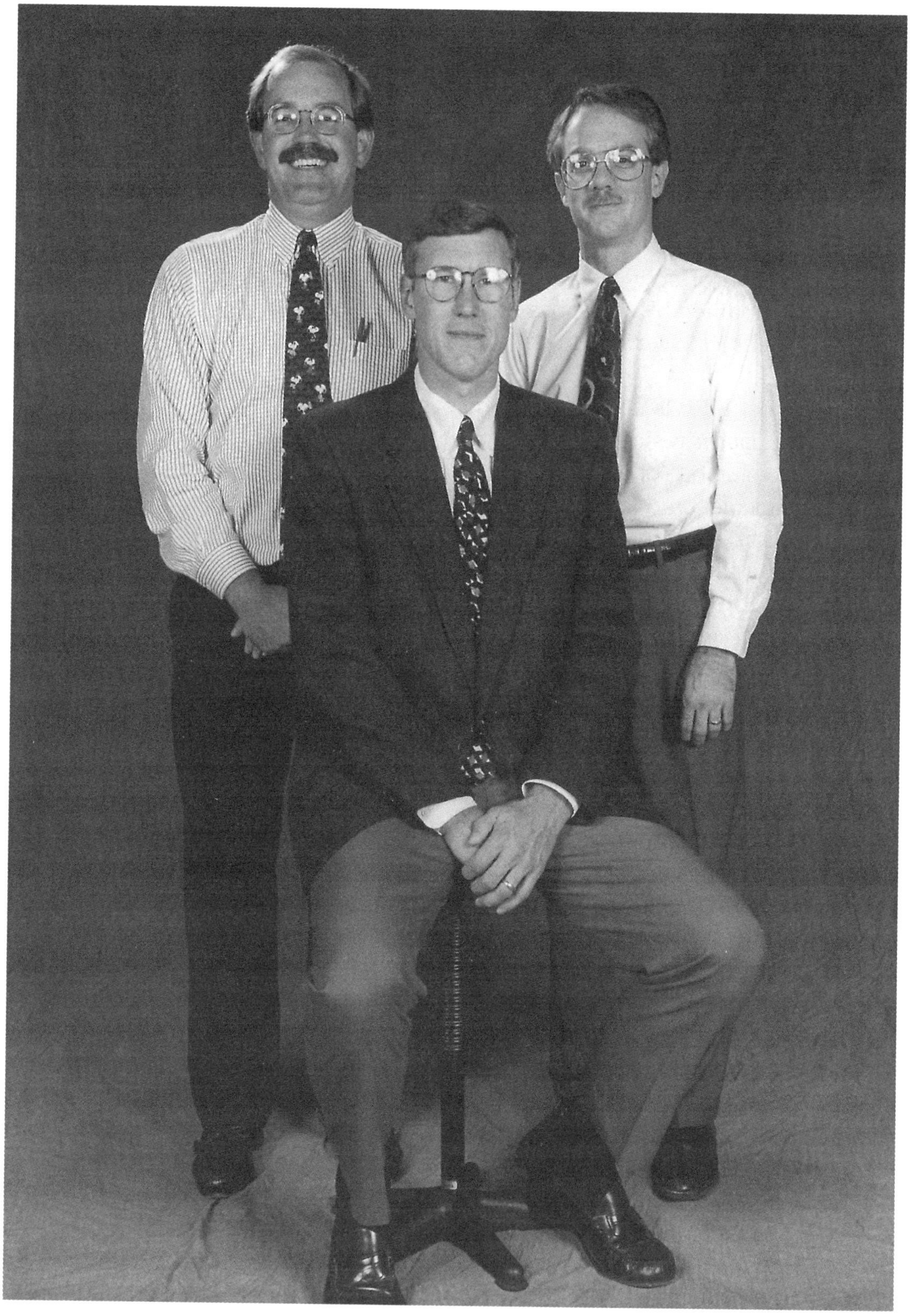

Children's Hospital Medical Center of Akron's orthopaedic staff. Left to right: Pat Riley, M.D., William Schrader, M.D., Paul Fleissner, Jr., M.D.

Children's Hospital Medical Center of Akron.

Chapter Five

Having their Say:

The preceding four chapters cover a century of scientific medical progress as shown in the development of Akron's orthopaedic residencies. In this chapter, eleven alumni of these programs have their say. Six attending orthopaedists from the third generation of teachers — Robert H. Bell, Gordon L. Bennett, J. Whit Ewing, Mark C. Leeson, Thomas J. Reilly, and Dennis S. Weiner tell how their subspecialties developed and how each became part of the Rubber City's orthopaedic armamentarium. In the second section, five recent graduates (1993 and 1996) — Drew R. Engles, Gerald Lang, Mark Peterson, Thomas Teater, and Matthew J. Weresh — reflect on their resident years.

Shoulder: The Akron Experience

by

Robert H. Bell, M.D.

Back as far as records of orthopaedic procedures go, there has always been a mystique surrounding the shoulder. Often the forgotten joint, owing in part to its complexity and difficulties of rehabilitation, the shoulder was, until the early 1980's, an area of only occasional scholarly efforts. Dr. Charles Neer, the preeminent investigator in this field, had done a number of retrospective clinical studies of various afflictions, such as rotator cuff tears and humeral fractures. Likewise, Dr. Carter Rowe of Boston had shown us the efficacy of the Bankart repair for anterior shoulder instability.

However, it was not until the late 1970's and early 1980's that the orthopaedic community truly began to demonstrate a sustained interest in this joint. It was during this time that Drs. Neer, Rowe, Rockwood, and Neviaser began to pollinate orthopaedics with their newly trained fellows, individuals who would one day themselves become the "young lions" of this new field of shoulder surgery. Their names are familiar now to us all: Matsen, Cofield, and Hawkins. To a man, they embodied many of the inherent strengths of their mentors, their academic curiosity and love of teaching, as well as their keen interest in exploring the surgical frontiers of this relatively unknown joint. These leaders provided the foundation upon which has been built not only the Shoulder and Elbow Society but, more importantly, the impetus for the sustained growth and interest in this area.

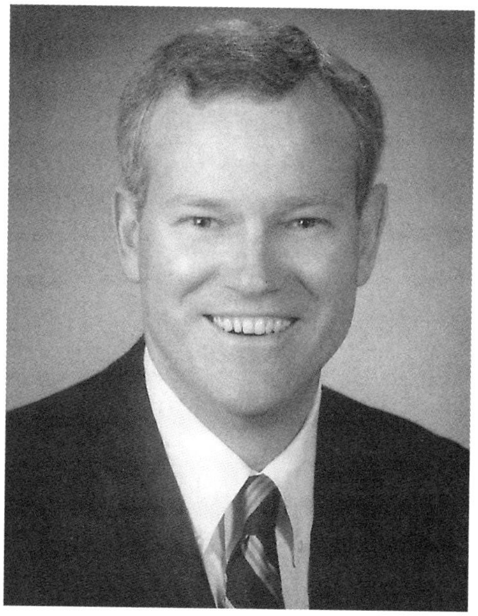

Robert H. Bell, M.D.

How then does Akron, Ohio, fit into this history? In order to understand the evolution of shoulder care in this community, one needs to travel back fifteen or twenty years. Repairs of the rotator cuff and Mumford procedures were the norm and represented the majority of surgical procedures. Instability was routinely addressed with either a Bristow or Magnuson-Stack procedure. Neer had recently published his report on the use of a humeral prosthesis for the treatment of complex fractures, and his concept of impingement and the efficacy of a limited acromioplasty versus an acromionectomy was being applied. Shoulder arthroscopy was but a twinkle in the eye of a few nationally known knee arthroscopists. One of these, prominent in the development of knee arthroscopy, was our own Whit Ewing.

It was in the early 1980's that things truly began to evolve. Whit, being a leader in the arthroscopic revolution, was performing up to thirty diagnostic knee arthroscopies a week. His patients, for the most part, came from referring orthopaedists for a diagnostic scope and then returned to them for a definitive arthrotomy and meniscectomy. It was not until 1981-82 that Whit began to routinely perform an arthroscopic partial meniscectomy. No one could have foreseen the enormous impact of this technological advance on the state of orthopaedics. General orthopaedists clamored to learn the new technique. At first somewhat reticent, fearing the new procedure was a victory of technology over reason, they slowly realized arthroscopy's potential to decrease morbidity and hospitalization with the potential for more rapid rehabilitation. The Age of Arthroscopy was born and with it came the realization that this tool could also be applied to other joints. Enter the shoulder.

As a young resident, coming upon my fifth and final year of training at Akron City Hospital, I was becoming increasingly aware of the growing interest in and need for subspecialization within orthopaedics. This change from the generalist to the specialist was not new to medicine or orthopaedics, but had previously been confined to the areas of hand, spine, and pediatric orthopaedics. Times were changing. The public was becoming increasingly more aware of, and educated in, the nuances of medicine and this was no different in our field.

Faced with the choice of becoming another general orthopaedist and possibly removing myself from the teaching and educational arena, I decided that subspecialization was my fate. At the same time, I was honored by a job offer from Dr. Hoyt and his group, Orthopaedic Surgeons, Inc. (now Crystal Clinic). After much consternation and some careful consideration, I chose to pursue a long unsatisfied interest in the area of the shoulder and elbow. I was fortunate to secure a six-month fellowship with Dr. Rich Hawkins, then one of the bright young leaders in the field of shoulder surgery.

I returned to Akron in January 1985 to embark on my new practice. Early on, it was apparent that the fastest growing area of interest within the field of shoulder and elbow surgery was that of arthroscopy, especially with the advent of Dr. Harvard Ellman's description of an arthroscopically performed acromioplasty. Unfortunately, I had only a limited amount of arthroscopic experience while with Dr. Hawkins and, consequently, I realized that self-teaching was to be my chosen route. With the encouragement of Whit Ewing and the group, my experience rapidly grew. Within two to three years I was performing one hundred to 120 arthroscopic acromioplasties annually.

Today, twelve years removed from that first year of frustration and learning, I find my practice slowly being overtaken by arthroscopic applications. Owing to the advent of new suture anchor devices and biodegradable tissue fixation tacks, many instability repairs are performed arthroscopically, as are many of the smaller rotator cuff repairs. Synovectomies, acromioclavicular joint excisions, and capsular releases are all commonplace. The improved rehabilitation, rapid return of motion, and patient satisfaction associated with these applications clearly demonstrate the efficacy of arthroscopy in shoulder problems.

Aside from the many new and exciting avenues of arthroscopy, the return of a number of other young, fellowship-trained men has provided the Akron community with a new perspective on this once forgotten joint. From shoulder and elbow arthroplasty to capsular shifts and supracapsular nerve decompressions, the shoulder has entered into the new age of orthopaedics in the Akron community. We are all privileged to be a part of this exciting renaissance.

Foot and Ankle Surgery in Akron

by

Gordon L. Bennett, M.D.

Although many area orthopaedic surgeons managed foot and ankle problems, no one claimed to have a subspecialty interest in foot and ankle until Mayo Clinic orthopaedist Dr. Kenneth Johnson came to Akron as the

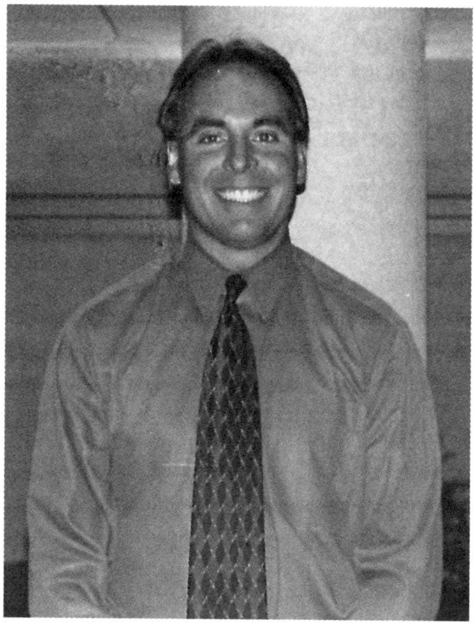

Gordon L. Bennett, M.D.

1985 Fowler B. Roberts Visiting Professor. A nationally and internationally renowned expert in foot and ankle disorders at the time, Dr. Johnson conducted one of the few fellowships in that subspecialty.

Dr. Johnson's two-day lectureship was extremely well received and stimulated significant interest in a variety of foot and ankle problems, including bunions and forefoot disorders, posterior tibial tendon dysfunction, and the multiply operated foot. It was not by chance that shortly after Dr. Johnson's visit, several Akron orthopaedic residents became interested in foot and ankle surgery and pursued fellowships in that subspecialty.

Since then, six Akron orthopaedic residents have done post-residency fellowships in foot and ankle reconstructive surgery. Three of these physicians currently practice in Akron and are actively involved in the orthopaedic surgery residency programs. State-of-the-art orthopaedic foot and ankle training is available to the orthopaedic residents in both programs.

Ian Alexander, M.D. (University of Western Ontario) came to Akron, Ohio in 1990. He had completed a one-year fellowship at the Mayo Clinic in Rochester, Minnesota under the direction of Dr. Kenneth Johnson and was in practice at the Cleveland Clinic Foundation prior to relocating to Akron. Dr. Alexander returned to Akron's Crystal Clinic after a sabbatical.

Gordon Bennett, M.D. (Akron General Medical Center-1988) completed a one-year fellowship at the University of Texas Southwestern Medical School in Dallas, Texas under the direction of Charles Graham, M.D. and Donald Mauldin, M.D. He was in practice in Vancouver, British Columbia, Canada for two years and returned to Akron in 1991. The majority of his practice involves foot and ankle care. He is an associate editor of *The Foot and Ankle International Journal.*

David Kay, M.D. (Akron General Medical Center-1986) completed a fellowship with F. William Wagner, M.D. at the University of Southern California in Los Angeles, California. He returned to Akron in 1987 and has been in practice since that time with a large majority of his practice devoted to foot and ankle care. He is an associate editor of *The Foot and Ankle International Journal.*

Harold Kitaoka, M.D. (Akron City Hospital-1986) completed a one-year fellowship at the University of California-Los Angeles Medical Center under the direction of Andrea Cracciola, M.D. He accepted a position at the Mayo Clinic in Rochester, Minnesota in 1987 and has been in practice there since that time. He is an associate editor of *The Foot and Ankle Journal*.

Christopher Klonk, M.D. (Akron City Hospital-1992) completed a six-month fellowship under the direction of Ian Alexander, M.D. in Akron, Ohio. He joined Orthopaedic Surgeons, Inc. (Crystal Clinic) in 1993 and devotes most of his practice to foot and ankle problems.

Thomas Krupko, M.D. (Akron City Hospital-1986) completed a six-month fellowship with James Sammarco, M.D. in Cincinnati, Ohio. He returned to Akron and practiced with the Falls Orthopaedic Group. He relocated to Alliance, Ohio, and is currently in practice in that location.

Steven Pearson, M.D. (Akron General Medical Center-1987) completed a one-year fellowship at the University of California-Los Angeles Medical Center under the direction of Andrea Cracciola, M.D. He went into private practice in Santa Barbara, California in 1988 and is still in that area.

Arthroscopy: Historical Perspectives and the Development of Arthroscopic Surgery in Akron, Ohio

by

J. W. Ewing, M.D.

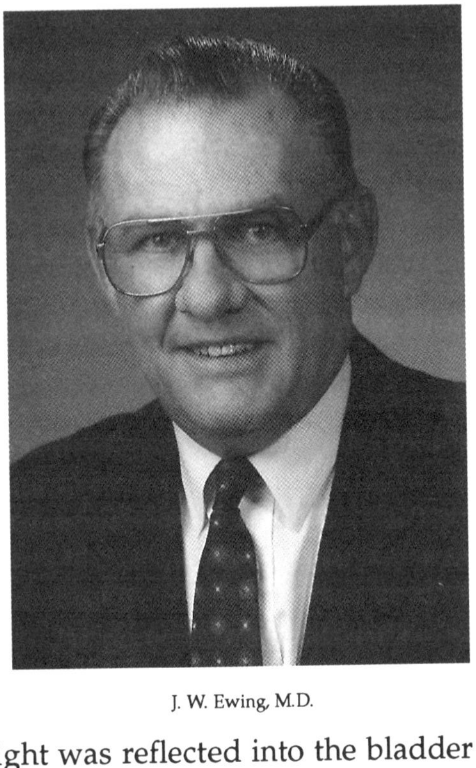

J. W. Ewing, M.D.

The earliest evidence of man's desire to explore the interior of body cavities is documented by references to vaginal specula in the ancient Hebrew literature and by the discovery of proctoscopes in the ruins of Pompeii. The bladder has been the most intriguing organ and has provided the major incentive in the development of endoscopic devices. The "Lichleiter," developed in 1806 by Botzini, was presented to the Joseph Academy of Medical Surgery, but the concept was not well received. The device consisted of two tubes and a candle as a light source. The light was reflected into the bladder of a patient through one tube, while the surgeon looked into the bladder through the other tube. Desormaux produced the gazogene endocystoscope in 1853. A mixture of turpentine and alcohol was used to provide the fuel for a fire in a small combustion chamber. The light from this fire was transmitted by way of mirrors into the bladder through a fairly large tube, which was also used for visualization. Max Nitze developed the first modern cystoscope in 1876. A platinum loop, heated by electricity and encased in a water cooled goose quill, provided the light source within the bladder. Finally, in 1880, Edison developed the incandescent lamp, which solved the problems of illumination and proved to be a milestone in the science of endoscopy. Cystoscopy then grew rapidly, and arthroscopy (the exploration of joint cavities) was a natural evolution.

Professor Kenji Takagi of Tokyo University is given credit for being the first to apply the principles of endoscopy successfully to a knee joint. Using a cystoscope, he viewed the interior of a cadaver knee in 1918. The stimulus for his work was the abundance of tuberculosis of the knee joint, which left the knee in a ankylosed condition. A Japanese citizen who can neither kneel nor squat has a serious physical as well as social disability. Takagi had hoped to diagnose tuberculosis arthritis early and provide more appropriate treatment. In 1919, he used a 7.3 mm arthroscope. In 1931, the #1 Takagi arthroscope was available. In 1932, he presented the first report of this instrument to the Japanese Orthopaedic Association in Tokyo. His report was accompanied by black and white photographs taken through the arthroscope. In 1936, he was successful in producing color photographs and a movie film.

World War II disrupted further advances in this science for a time. Following the war, Dr. Masaki Watanabe, a student of Professor Takagi, continued his work. In 1958, he released the Watanabe #21. It proved to be the first truly successful arthroscope. This instrument had a depth of focus from 0.5 mm to infinity. The lenses were hand ground by a craftsman named Fukuyo. An incandescent bulb that protruded slightly beyond the end of the arthroscope provided the illumination necessary for visualization.

Cold light provided by fiber optics was the next major advance in the development of the arthroscope. This advance led to the development of smaller arthroscopes, such as the Watanabe #24, which was only 2 mm in diameter. Dr. Watanabe performed his first arthroscopic meniscectomy on May 4, 1962. In 1957, the first edition of Watanabe's *Atlas of Arthroscopy* was published. This atlas was revised and republished in 1969. It contained actual photographs of joint pathology.

In Europe, Dr. Eugen Bircher introduced the Jacobeus laparoscope into the knee in 1921. He called the technique "arthro-endoscopy." Bircher used carbon dioxide to distend the joint, and described post traumatic arthritis and ruptured menisci in articles published in 1921 and 1922.

Dr. Phillip Kreuscher published the first United States article on this procedure in 1925. His article appeared in the *Illinois Medical Journal.* In 1930, Dr. Michael Burman, of New York's Hospital for Joint Diseases, spent a fellowship year in Germany studying endoscopic techniques. He returned to the States and, using cadaver specimens, arthroscoped every joint in the body. Burman published several articles on this new method of examining joints, but his methods were met with skepticism by the orthopaedic community. Arthroscopy remained absent from the scene in the United States until the 1960's.

Thanks to Dr. Robert Jackson from Toronto, Ontario, Canada for re-introducing arthroscopy to North America. Dr. Jackson went to Tokyo University in 1964 with the main purpose of studying tissue culture techniques. While there, he met Dr. Watanabe and observed arthroscopic techniques. He returned to Toronto in 1965 and began to practice arthroscopy using the Watanabe #21 arthroscope. In 1967, he gave a presentation on the subject of arthroscopy at the Association of Academic Surgeons meeting, held in Toronto. In 1968, Dr. Jackson gave the first instructional course dealing with arthroscopy at the American Academy of Orthopaedic Surgeons meeting. Virtually no other surgeons in North America were practicing arthroscopy at that time.

Interest rapidly grew from the point of re-introduction of the technique by Dr. Jackson. Early contributors from those days in the late sixties and early seventies include people such as Dr. Ward Cassells, Dr. Jack McGinty, Dr. Bob Metcalf, Dr. John Joyce, Dr. Ken Dehaven, and others. In 1969, Dr. Richard O'Conner, from West Covina, California, visited Dr. Watanabe and soon began to develop techniques for meniscal surgery.

In 1972, the International Arthroscopy Association was founded in Philadelphia. Professor Watanabe was elected the first chairman. The purpose of the organization was to educate orthopaedic surgeons to the value of the technique and to spread awareness of arthroscopy to all parts of the world. Numerous courses were developed from that point in time and arthroscopy grew rapidly. The first major course in the United States was given at the University of Pennsylvania under the chairmanship of Dr. John Joyce. Over the next decade, literally hundreds of arthroscopic courses were held throughout the world and more and more orthopaedists became aware of the potential for this way of approaching joint pathology. In 1982, the Arthroscopy Association of North America was founded. It is now the largest such Association in the world.

Arthroscopy in Akron began at City Hospital in 1972. The first arthroscope brought into the hospital was a Watanabe #26 model purchased by Dr. Whit Ewing. He had read the *Atlas of Arthroscopy* by Dr. Watanabe and was intrigued by what seemed to him to be the logical way to establish a correct diagnosis of knee joint pathology. At that time, there were no practical courses that offered hands-on teaching of this skill. Dr. Ewing took time from the practice of general orthopaedics and developed his techniques for arthroscopy using cadavers available to him in the autopsy room at Akron City Hospital. He was encouraged by his associates in practice and, in particular, by his mentor, Dr. Walter A. Hoyt, Jr. He arthroscoped nearly all the joints in the body over a several month period of time, but concentrated on the knee joint.

The first clinical trial of arthroscopy at Akron City Hospital was carried out in January 1973. In that particular case, what seemed to be a clear cut bucket handle tear of the medial meniscus, turned out to be a torn lateral meniscus instead. That first case, where a young athlete was spared an inappropriate medial arthrotomy, was enough to enflame the young doctor's enthusiasm. Drs. Herbert Thompson and George Mallo began to apply the techniques of diagnostic arthroscopy to their patients at about the same time, and were equally convinced of the validity of the technique. Many members of the orthopaedic staff at Akron City Hospital began to ask Dr. Ewing to arthroscope their patients as a means of diagnostic consultation. These patients had their knees arthroscoped under local anesthesia, then were returned to their orthopaedist for definitive care. This is just one example of the closely knit staff that existed at City and persists at the Summa Health System program.

Dr. Ewing held the first regional arthroscopy course at the Kent Holiday Inn in 1979. That meeting sold out. Drs. Bob Metcalf, Bob Eilert, and Lanny Johnson joined Dr. Ewing on the faculty. By this time, arthroscopic partial meniscectomies were routinely being taught in the residency program by a number of the staff at City Hospital. Very few university programs had even begun to perform arthroscopy as yet. Akron City Hospital had become recognized nationally as a teaching center of arthroscopic surgery within its already highly regarded program of orthopaedic surgery. Numerous instruments used daily thoughout the world were developed with input from City Hospital. Many published articles and book chapters have emanated from the staff as well. Dr. Ewing headed the education committee of the Arthroscopy Association of North America for five years in the eighties and became president of that organization in 1992.

Arthoscopic surgical procedures now make up the majority of elective orthopaedic procedures done by the orthopaedic department at Summa Health System hospitals. The orthopaedic staff now has surgeons routinely doing ligament reconstructions, rotator cuff tears, shoulder stabilizations, ankle debridements, wrist arthroscopy, and elbow arthroscopy. Current clinical and basic research in arthroscopy continues actively. Equipped with the latest arthroscopic equipment available, the department continues to serve the citizens of Akron and the surrounding communities with the confident skill of people who know what they are doing and who continue to seek better ways of doing it.

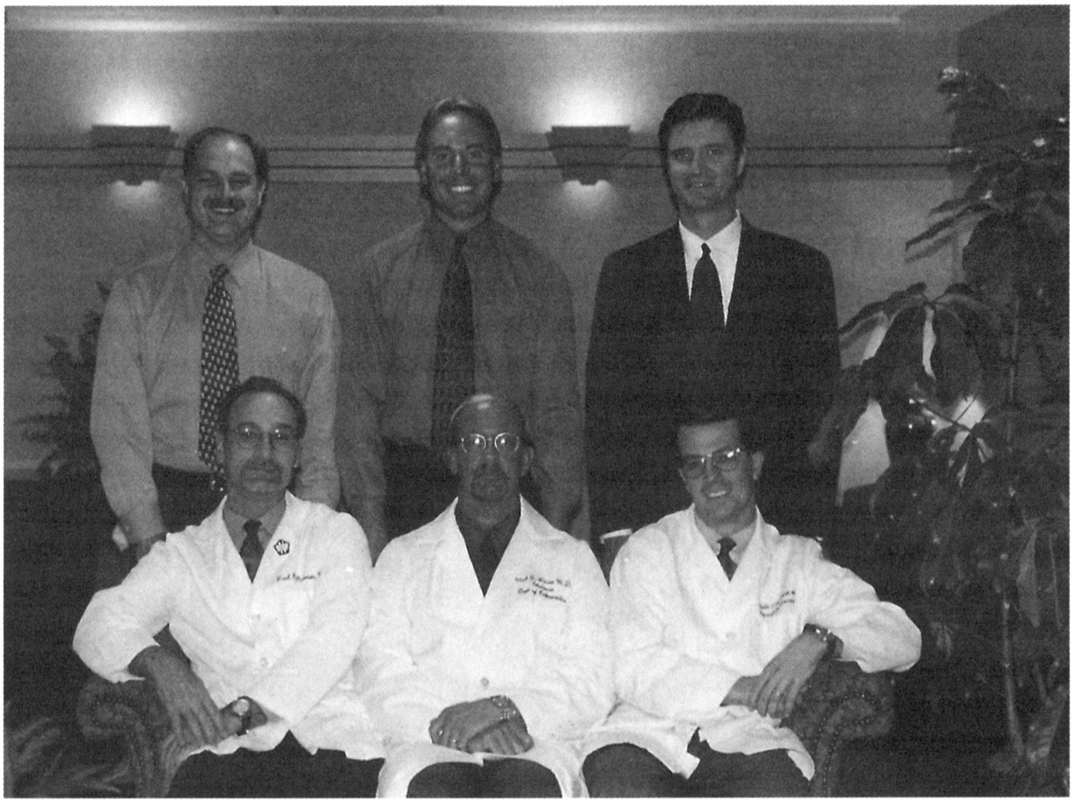

Akron General Medical Center Staff -- Faculty of AGMC's orthopaedic residency program. Left to right -- Back Row: Gregory Vrabec, Gordon Bennett, Michael Smith. Left to right -- Front Row: Paul Reiman, Mark Leeson, and Michael Prayson.

Photo by Penny La Bate

Orthopaedic Oncology in Akron

by

Mark C. Leeson, M.D.

Orthopaedic oncology is the care and treatment of patients, both pediatric and adult, with musculoskeletal neoplasms (benign and/or malignant, primary and/or metastatic) which involve the musculoskeletal system (bone, muscle, tendon, joint, etc.).

Orthopaedic oncology (although not by name) has been discussed in some of the most ancient writings available regarding medicine. Hippocrates described patients with metastatic disease or malignant tumors of bone and muscle, as did other prominent writers of medical literature in ancient Greece and Rome.

In the mythology of ancient Rome, there is a very prominent myth regarding the resection or amputation of the diseased limb and transplantation (with an allograft) from a twin brother's limb. This was the first known description or discussion of an allograft transplantation.

The availability of the x-ray or roentgen first allowed physicians to see and then describe radiographic abnormalities associated with or caused by neoplastic conditions. In the early and middle part of the twentieth century, as the use of x-rays and the microscope became more common, a number of centers began to describe, discuss, and classify neoplastic conditions of bone and muscle.

One of the first series written about patients treated with orthopaedic oncologic procedures was published in the 1920's. An orthopaedic surgeon named Dr. Lexer described the removal of diseased or neoplastic bone and replacement with fresh allograft bone. Despite this early scholarly activity, orthopaedic oncology was still in its embryonic phase. The development of chemotherapy in the 1960's allowed patients to have earlier and more aggressive treatment (usually for metastatic conditions). The treatment of primary neoplastic conditions involving the bone and muscle was usually amputation and the results were often dismal for the patient and discouraging for the surgeon.

In Akron before the 1980's, physicians made sporadic operative reports about patients who were treated for oncologic conditions with resections, amputations, and a wide assortment of operative procedures, but there is little good historical data prior to 1980 with regard to the incidence of conditions such as osteogenic sarcoma, Ewing's sarcoma, myeloma, or even metastatic disease involving bone. In the mid-1970's, Dr. John W. Ewing had some interest in orthopaedic oncology and saw a number of patients for both benign and malignant conditions and attempted to improve the care delivered locally to patients with these problems. In 1984, Dr. Mark C. Leeson returned from a fellowship in orthopaedic oncology as the first fellowship-trained orthopaedic oncologist in the Akron area. He also was named Director of Resident Education and Research at Akron General Medical Center, but provided orthopaedic oncologic care to patients in all hospitals and throughout the region.

The ability to use the bone scan, the CAT scan, and the advent of the MRI scan have greatly aided and improved the early evaluation and diagnosis of patients with musculoskeletal neoplasms. Early diagnosis and appropriate and aggressive multi-specialty treatment have greatly improved the prognosis for most patients with these often devastating problems. Dr. Mark Leeson and Dr. David Kay were the first physicians in Ohio to apply an Ilizarov external fixator for the lengthening of osteogenesis of bone. While this was not used in this particular case for a tumor, it has been used since in the treatment of patients with neoplastic conditions very successfully.

Along with the improvement in scanning and radiographic techniques has come the ability to use other reconstructive measures as well. Two main treatments used in the reconstruction for patients with oncologic problems are mega-prostheses (often customized, made with metal such as titanium or alloys) and large allograft bone. Often a combination of "devices" is used for reconstructive purposes.

The goal has been to diminish local recurrence, improve long-term survival, and provide function without the necessity of an amputation. This has been extremely successful. Among the first one hundred of Dr. Leeson's patients with primary soft tissue sarcomas (muscle, tendon, etc.), only one required an amputation. Of the first one hundred patients treated by Dr. Leeson who did not have a biopsy or previous treatment done elsewhere, local recurrence was less than 2 percent and survival at five years was approximately 93 percent. Even young children with catastrophic diseases such as Ewing's sarcoma and osteogenic sarcoma are often treated today with neoadjuvant chemotherapy, local resection, and reconstructive procedures, with diminished local recurrence and dramatically improved long-term survival.

Orthopaedic oncology has become a complex field which requires an inter-disciplinary team approach in many instances. We have become very fortunate in the Akron area to have exceptional, fellowship-trained individuals to assist with radiation oncology and medical oncology (the administration and management of chemotherapeutic agents).

We (collectively as a community) are active members in multiple onologic groups, such as the Children's Cancer Study Group, the Inner Group for Ewing's, the Eastern Oncologic Group, the Southwest Oncologic Group, etc. Being members of so many large and important multi-institutional groups allows us in Akron to administer up-to-the-minute, state-of-the-art, multi-disciplinary approaches and treatments for all patients with neoplastic conditions. Dr. Leeson, who is now Chairman of the Department of Orthopaedic Surgery at Akron General Medical Center, is also a member of the Musculoskeletal Tumor Society and the Society of Surgical Oncology, and has been an active presenter of research to both of these groups.

Research in the area of orthopaedic oncology has also been active in Akron. Beginning in 1984, with Dr. Leeson's return, approximately fifteen to twenty research projects have been completed and presented locally, nationally, and internationally. A large number have also been published in refereed journals. Orthopaedic oncologic research done in Akron has been presented by Dr. Leeson in Kyoto, Japan, St. Malo, France, Bologna, Italy, Montreal, Canada, and throughout the United States. In 1989, Dr. Leeson was also awarded the Mid-America Orthopaedic Association Travelling Fellowship, which he took in the area of orthopaedic oncology.

By 1994, Dr. Leeson had treated more than 2,500 patients with neoplastic conditions, both benign and malignant, primary and metastatic, with impressively successful results here in Akron, Ohio. In 1992, Dr. Scott Weiner returned from a fellowship at the University of Florida to work at Summa Health System in the area of orthopaedic oncology, trauma, and resident basic science education.

It is safe to say, from very humble beginnings, that we have developed a "center of excellence" in orthopaedic oncology here in Akron that allows us to provide state-of-the-art care for patients, both locally and as a tertiary referral center.

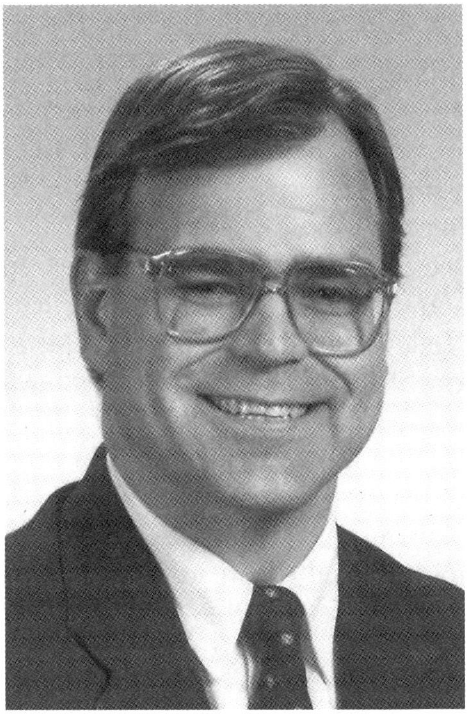

Thomas J. Reilly, M. D.

"On the Shoulders of Giants" Hand Surgery in Akron, Ohio

by

Thomas J. Reilly, M.D.

In 1675, Sir Isaac Newton said, "If I have seen further...it is from standing on the shoulders of giants." Dr. Joseph Boyes titled his book *On the Shoulders of Giants* to give credit to the "giants" in history who have contributed to our current knowledge of hand surgery.

Orthopaedics in Akron very much parallels the development of hand surgery as a specialty. The American Society for Surgery of the Hand was founded in 1946 by Sterling Bunnell, the same year the orthopaedic residency was established at City Hospital. Hand surgery as a specialty grew in Akron as hand surgery as a specialty grew nationally.

In 1947, after a nine month internship and three months of orthopaedic residency, Dr. William Davis found himself a first lieutenant in California. He was assigned to work as a resident on the trauma service at Letterman General Hospital in San Francisco. Every Tuesday afternoon, Dr. Davis first-assisted a noted surgeon named Sterling Bunnell. This experience, one year after the founding of the American Society for Surgery of the Hand and the orthopaedic residency in Akron, Dr. Davis brought back to Akron. He began building the solid foundation that enabled hand surgery to grow as a specialty in Akron at the same pace that hand surgery grew in the United States.

In the 1950's in Akron, the rubber industry was booming. The automobile industry also found northeast Ohio to be a favorable environment for growth and production. It was this industrial base that provided Akron orthopaedic hand surgeons exposure to complex hand trauma. Dr. Davis worked closely with the plant physicians at Chrysler's Twinsburg plant to help make the stamping machines safer. At that time as many as ten press injuries a week would present to City Hospital alone.

At the 1962 national meeting of the American Society for Surgery of the Hand in Miami, Florida, Dr. Adrian Flatt presented his experience with prosthetic replacements of arthritic joints of the hand. Traditional teaching at that time was not to operate on the joints of a rheumatoid because you "would only make things worse." In 1963, Dr. William Davis and an orthopaedic resident, Douglas Corwin, visited Dr. Flatt in Iowa City. Dr. Flatt did four cases that day. The visitors from Ohio watched the first two cases and then, to their surprise, Dr. Flatt asked Dr. Davis to assist on the third case and Doug Corwin on the fourth case! Dr. Flatt and Dr. Sterling Bunnell, giants of hand surgery, obviously, directly contributed to our knowledge here in Akron.

Formal training in hand surgery was not common prior to the 1960's. Surgeons who pursued their interest in surgery of the hand were mostly self-taught through attending meetings and personal communications. Primary flexor tendon surgery in zone two was fraught with complications. Verdan presented his technique of primary repair with satisfactory results. Shortly after this, Dr. Davis was performing flexor tendon repairs in selected patients on a primary basis.

The transition to our next "giant" began in an interesting way. In 1965, Dr. Davis performed the first microscopic digital nerve repair in Akron. The patient was injured in a work related accident. The microscope from Dr. Falor's research lab was used and "delicate" 7-0 silk sutures reapproximated the digital nerve. Although the operating room surgeon reports that two point discrimination is normal, those of us who followed our training in Akron are all fortunate that the nerve that was cut was the ulnar digital nerve on Dr. Tom Reef's middle finger. The laceration occurred in surgery when Dr. Reef was cut with a scalpel. He recovered not only to finish his residency, but to become the first Akron resident to pursue a year of formal training in hand surgery.

Tom Reef spent twelve months in New York under the direction of Dr. William Littler, another founding member of the American Society for Surgery of the Hand. When Dr. Reef returned to Akron he practiced hand surgery as well as general orthopaedics. After one year, however, he made the bold step of going out on his own to limit his practice to surgery of the hand. Tom's practice was the foundation for the current Summit Hand Center group in Akron, which has now grown to five physicians.

Throughout the 1970's, hand surgery became more recognized as a specialty nationally. Microvascular replantation was introduced in the late 1960's and 1970's as a technique to reattach amputated digits and extremities. Dr. Frank Forshew brought this technology back to northeast Ohio when he returned from his fellowships with Harold Kleinert and Joe Kutz in Louisville, Kentucky, and Dr. Adrian Flatt in Iowa. When Frank returned in 1975, he joined Tom Reef in practice to form the first hand surgery group in Ohio.

Over the next twenty years hand surgery continued to grow, contributing to advanced care for patients as well as education of residents here in Akron. Major limb replantation and digital replantation became commonplace and Akron became a regional referral center for major hand trauma. Today, patients travel to Akron for hand care from up to two hours away. Half our patients are from outside Summit County.

In 1984, a young boy presented to Dr. Dennis Weiner at Children's Hospital with complaints of left shoulder pain. Evaluation revealed a suspicious lytic defect in the child's proximal humerus. This young boy truly represents what is great and unique about the Akron orthopaedic community. Dr. Weiner consulted Dr. Mark Leeson, who had recently returned to Akron, having completed a fellowship in orthopaedic oncology. Biopsy proved the diagnosis of osteosarcoma and a radical, but limb sparing resection was carried out. Dr. Leeson then collaborated with the hand service to assist in limb salvage reconstruction. T.J. Reilly was in the midst of his fellowship at Louisville where research was being carried out on osteocutaneous, vascular fibula transfers. T.J. made a January return to Akron where, in a fourteen-hour operation, he teamed with Dr. Leeson and Dr. Forshew to restore this young boy's proximal humerus with a vascularized fibula. Eleven years later this young boy not only is alive, but has a functioning upper extremity that gives him no difficulties. Cooperation between orthopaedists, between hospitals, and between subspecialists allowed a truly remarkable recovery for this young boy. Since 1985, the vascularized fibula has been utilized over thirty times for limb salvage here in Akron. Most recently, a one-year-old boy, patient of Dr. Dennis Weiner and Dr. Bill Schrader, with congenital pseudoarthrosis of the tibia, having failed traditional bone grafting, has healed his tibia, following vascularized fibula transfer.

In 1985, Akron lost one of its "giants," Tom Reef, at the young age of forty-nine to colon cancer. T.J. Reilly returned to town to work with Dr. Forshew. Dr. Nina Njus came from Iowa to join Summit Hand Center in 1986. Shortly after this, Dr. Bill McCue limited his practice to surgery of the hand and also joined the group. Dr. John Dietrich and Dr. John Biondi also brought expertise from their fellowship programs in Pittsburgh and Loma Linda respectively, to northeast Ohio.

Tragedy returned to the orthopaedic community in March of 1992 when Frank Forshew was killed in a place crash as he was returning from a meeting. The tragic loss of Frank and Tom at the peaks of their careers emphasized their great contributions to development of hand surgery here in Akron. Those of us who benefitted from their teaching as well as the countless number of patients who benefitted from their experience will be forever grateful.

Over fifty years of hand surgery in the United States parallels the growth of orthopaedics and hand surgery here in Akron. We are indebted to the giants of hand surgery that have proceeded us and to their dedication to hand surgery as a specialty. They have left us with a legacy. That legacy is to continue to educate our residents and our medical colleagues, as well as provide the highest quality of specialty hand care for our patients.

Children's Hospital Medical Center of Akron
Its Role in Orthopaedic Surgery in the Community

by

Dennis S. Weiner, M.D.

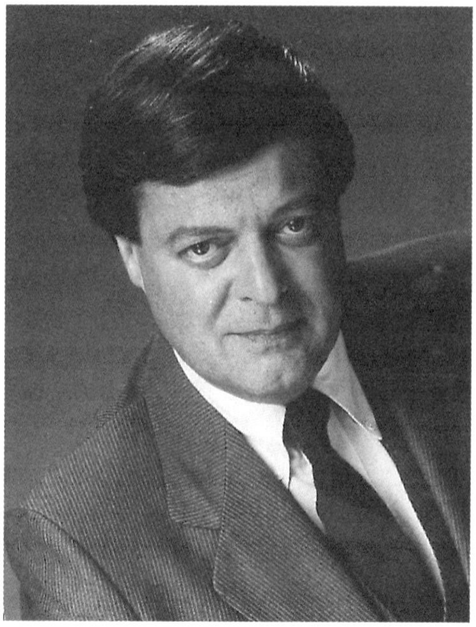

Dennis S. Weiner, M. D.

The Akron Day Nursery was established in 1890 to care for children whose mothers worked outside the home. Sponsors added a Ward for Crippled Children in 1905. By 1910, the Nursery had evolved into the Mary Day Nursery and Children's Hospital. In 1918, Akron Children's Hospital's Orthopaedic Clinic opened under the leadership of Walter A. Hoyt, Sr., M.D. The clinic flourished, tripling in size in one year.

A special clinic for polio (infantile paralysis) opened in 1918 and Children's orthopaedists diagnosed forty-two cases of the disease that year. The State of Ohio, through its Department of Charities, chose Akron Children's Hospital as one of eight orthopaedic centers in Ohio in 1921. In 1922, over 2,800 patients were seen at the Orthopaedic Clinic. It was estimated then that, under the auspices of the Ohio Society for Crippled Children, the hospital would care for as many as two thousand children with polio from eight northeastern Ohio counties.

Infantile paralysis, or polio, was, without question, the dominant condition treated at the hospital for the next forty years. Children with orthopaedic handicaps were hospitalized for long periods of time, which led to concern over educational deficiencies. A 1921 grant from the Ohio State

Educational Department provided a teacher for in-hospital schooling.

By 1935, the Department of Orthopaedics consisted of three members and two residents. The senior staff included Drs. Walter A. Hoyt, Sr., Fowler B. Roberts, and Harold Conn. Dr. Hoyt, Sr. and Dr. Adrian E. Davis, in association with a resident, Dr. George Van Buren, treated osteomyelitis patients with the new sulfa drugs in 1940.

It was estimated that roughly 10 to 15 percent of all polio victims seen at Children's required orthopaedic surgery. By 1940, three hundred patients had been seen with orthopaedic complications of infantile paralysis. In 1944, during a particularly heavy outbreak of polio, Children's Hospital was designated one of several Polio Centers for the State of Ohio, admitting approximately 20 percent of all polio patients in the state.

In 1947, the most severe epidemic yet struck Akron. By early autumn, 415 polio patients were hospitalized at Children's, with the neighboring Grace Evangelical and Reformed Church taking the hospital's overflow. (As a side note, I spent three weeks in the church as a polio patient and fortunately recovered well.) An even bigger outbreak occurred in 1952 and the patients in-house totalled over six hundred.

The twelve-bed surgical and orthopaedic ward was chronically full by 1948; an adolescent and orthopaedic ward of thirty-five beds opened in 1978. Dennis S. Weiner, M.D. eventually assumed the directorship of the Juvenile Amputee Clinic, which was established in 1965 under the guidance of Walter A. Hoyt, Jr., M.D. This clinic merged with our regular orthopaedic clinic in 1985.

In conjunction with Akron City Hospital, Dr. Walter A. Hoyt, Sr. and Dr. Fowler B. Roberts established the orthopaedic residency at Children's Hospital in 1946. For over forty years, Children's Department of Orthopaedics has operated field clinics to provide diagnostic and treatment services throughout much of the State of Ohio. These clinics began under the auspices of the Bureau of Crippled Children's Services, which is now the Bureau of Maternal and Child Health. Currently, orthopaedic clinics operate in the following Ohio cities — Dover, Alliance, Norwalk, Salem, Steubenville, and Martin's Ferry.

Research into pediatric orthopaedic conditions has been heavily emphasized at Children's since 1970 and has resulted in nearly one hundred publications, including a textbook on pediatric orthopaedics. The current staff includes four full-time pediatric surgeons, Drs. Dennis S. Weiner, Department Chairman and Director of Research, Patrick Riley, William Schrader, and Paul Fleissner. The Department of Orthopaedics at Children's Hospital Medical Center of Akron is recognized nationally for the high quality of its orthopaedic residency training program as well as its major contributions to our understanding of children's bone and joint diseases.

Residents Recall Their Training

Drew R. Engles, M.D., Akron General Medical Center, '96

When I was asked to comment on my experience as an orthopaedic surgery resident in Akron, Ohio, my thoughts immediately focused on what a special time this was in my life. I suspect as you read the essays of other Akron orthopaedic graduates you will find this was a universally important time for each of us, both in personal and professional growth. How then has Akron provided such a nurturing environment for future orthopaedists? I believe there are two reasons. First, orthopaedic surgery as a specialty, or better yet, as a calling, attracts a certain type of individual. Secondly, and perhaps more importantly, there has been an unbroken string of mentors who have devoted their lives to the postgraduate education of subsequent generations of orthopaedic surgeons.

Even as a naive medical student, I had an inkling of what separated orthopaedic surgeons from other physicians. The following paragraphs were my original thoughts during the arduous application process for an orthopaedic residency:

"Orthopaedic surgeons are *Iliad* people. When I was a junior in college, a professor of Greek literature digressed from the opus at hand one day to explain his view of the world. He said the planet could be divided into two types of people, *Odyssey* People and *Iliad* People. The *Odyssey* People were a contempletive lot who went through life pondering its many problems and complexities as they bumped into them. These individuals were not unlike Odysseus who meandered about the Mediterranean for a decade as he made his way back to Ithaca at the end of the Trojan War. They are thinkers and among their ranks are our philosophers and artists. At their best they are the world's greatest minds. At their worst they are miserable loners.

He also felt that Achilles, hero of the Homeric epic, was the icon for the rest of the world. *Iliad* People, as he called them, met the world head on. You could not explain a setback or failure to them. You were just describing a greater challenge. *Iliad* People, he said, were full of hubris, a Greek word best translated as self-confidence and pride. In singularity they could be stubborn. In unison they were overwhelming.

Orthopaedic surgeons are definitely *Iliad* People. I could see this from the first one I ever met and I was sure of it after the initial day of my junior clerkship in medical school. On the orthopaedic service, rounds went at a pace one notch above the rest in the hospital. Notes were succinct and problems were immediately addressed. There was a definite "roll up your sleeves and get to work" attitude present. There was, however, something else. There was a sense of camaraderie among the residents. I do not know if this was a function of personalities or purpose. As residents they seemed more content than their colleagues, not any less tired of health care bureaucracy, but perhaps more satisfied.

My classmates thought of orthopaedic surgery as a "fun rotation." I saw it as a career. In either case, there was little separating the two. The diversity in the age of the orthopaedic population, ranging from the infant to the geriatric, as well as the broad spectrum of pathology and severity of illness appealed to me. The singularity of purpose with which one heads to the operating room, the dexterity and expertise in anatomy required for success, and the satisfaction that one receives from the fruitful combination of these entities appealed to me."

While this may explain common bonds that link all orthopaedic surgeons, it does not fully explain the success or the unique atmosphere in Akron. The key rests in the endeavors of the men who have developed and led the orthopaedic programs in Akron.

At Akron City Hospital, the baton was passed from Dr. Walter Hoyt to Dr. J. Patrick Flanagan. Dr. Hoyt brought national recognition to Akron when he was elected president of the American Academy of Orthopaedic Surgeons. Today, Dr. Flanagan continues to strengthen the program by recruiting former graduates to return after they have acquired specialized training both nationally and abroad.

At Children's Hospital Medical Center of Akron, Dr. Dennis Weiner has been a fixture in the education of residents from both Akron and Cleveland. He has been a proponent and sponsor of resident research for years. More recently, the return to Northeast Ohio of both of Dr. Weiner's sons to practice is yet another testimony to the rich heritage of Akron orthopaedics.

At Akron General Medical Center, I had the privilege of being selected by Dr. Buel Smith. Having had the opportunity to survey residency programs across the United States and in Europe, I have yet to see an educational program that rivals the morning lecture schedule that was championed by Dr. Smith. While he will claim that it is the result of fine tuning by each group of residents year after year, we all see his gentle hand guiding the process. In addition, because of the overlap in careers, I was also afforded the opportunity to train under Dr. Harry O'Dell and Dr. Mark Leeson, Dr. Smith's predecessor and successor respectively. Each of these men has left an indelible mark on the residency program and on me. Dr. Smith instilled in each of us a certain tacit expectation to perform at a level above what had been asked of us. From Dr. O'Dell I learned that regardless of the situation, one can always remain a gentleman first and a surgeon second. Dr. Leeson provided a paradigm for remaining the sole unflustered individual when all around you are mired in a sea of turmoil.

It was an unparalleled educational opportunity to train in such an environment, a pleasure to live in the community, and it was an honor to be associated with the attendings and residents who cared for the injured at the hospitals of Akron, Ohio. To the aforementioned mentors, to whom we collectively owe a great debt of gratitude, I personally thank you.

Gerald J. Lang, M.D., City, '93

It is Match Day, March 15, 11am, at a midwestern medical school. My wife already has her envelope (we're in the couples match), but she is too chicken to open it. She insists that I open mine first. After a long wait, my name is called and I pick up my envelope. I open it...Orthopaedic Surgery, Akron City Hospital, Akron, Ohio! My immediate response is a combination of excitement and relief. The past six months of uncertainty had taken its toll. Matching in a very competitive field, in one of my preferred residency programs, was beyond my dreams.

Once I returned to reality, I anxiously awaited my wife's response. I could tell that she was somewhat pleased, but I knew she would have preferred to stay closer to home. She was happy that we would be at the same hospital during our residencies, but she was a little apprehensive about spending five years in a town known best for the Rubber Bowl and the Soap Box Derby. People in this town root for a color (Browns), part of a jacket (Zips), and a nut (Buckeyes).

Three months later, my wife and I traveled 500 miles to our new home. We settled in, survived the orientation process and anxiously began our internships. It became apparent that a lot of the stuff I learned in medical school was worth remembering. We became highly skilled at working long hours with very little sleep. You have to somehow convince yourself that this new found experience of working >100 hrs/wk is okay. I guess we just didn't know any better.

During my initial orthopaedic rotation, I had the honor of assisting on my first legimate orthopaedic case — a sliding hip screw, on a 90 y/o woman named Della. (How can you forget a name like that!) The chief resident had gone over things with me a few times beforehand. Things went as planned and the postoperative x-rays looked perfect. Little did I know that in a few short years, I would be taking an intern through his first case, just as the attending surgeon did with me.

As time passed, there were more patients, more cases, and many late nights in the emergency department. Rounds began early and surgeries ran late while clinic lists grew longer. People you worked with each day became your closest friends and support group. Sanity was preserved with the help of frequent gatherings on Wednesday nights at Cascade Park (soft ball) or Balch Street Gym (basketball). The Bell Volley Ball Open (BVO), St. Patrick's Day, and Post Grad Day always kept you going. Somehow, we made it through with very few casualties.

My educational endeavors carried me from San Francisco to Switzerland and many places in between. Lectures, courses, workshops, and visiting professors filled in the cracks on a busy schedule. Pat Flanagan and Co. have done a good job in preparing me for the future. I enjoy the luxury of having had a broad base of knowledge and experience which has served me well.

I have since left Akron, completed a fellowship, and returned closer to home. We left many close friends and good memories there. Akron is a special place that I visited at a special time in my life. It proved to be a very fertile environment for growth in my personal and professional life. My wife and I will always remember this early chapter in our lives and look back with fond memories.

Mark D. Peterson, M.D. City, '93

The efforts of many dedicated surgeons, some discussed in the preceding text and others not mentioned, have allowed fortunate individuals the opportunity to experience an extraordinary orthopaedic education. I am one of those fortunate individuals.

After rotating on orthopaedic services at three large universities and driving over two thousand miles as a visiting medical student from Oregon, Akron, Ohio seemed like a foreign country. This was not due to the distance I had traveled, but rather to the nature and quality of the education I encountered. The academic intensity, enthusiasm, and collegial spirit were almost unbelievable. How could this community based program in northeast Ohio have so much to offer? It took me several years to find the answer to this question.

Unlike many of the "best" orthopaedic training programs in the country, held at tertiary referral centers, Akron is on the "front line" of orthopaedic care and offers a tremendous exposure to common orthopaedic problems. However, like many large centers, Akron's staff includes fellowship trained subspecialists in nearly all areas of orthopaedics and serves as a referral center for many surrounding communities. This unique situation provides a rare balance of clinical material ideal for resident training. However, I do not believe this is the reason Akron orthopaedics is so special.

The first clue to the answer to my question was provided by Dr. Flanagan when discussing the expected performance of his new interns and residents: "good and excellent are acceptable, anything else gets a pink slip." These were horrifying words to a new intern, but I soon realized that they represented the philosophy that set Akron apart from other orthopaedic training programs.

A few years later, after a suspected trip to Mt. Sinai, Dr. Flanagan answered a little bit more of my question. "Care of the patient always comes first" was the first commandment of orthopaedics...it was also the second, third, fourth, and fifth commandments.

Many attendings and residents throughout my residency helped answer this question as well, through numerous outstanding lectures, superb surgical instruction, and research of the highest quality.

Other experiences, such as feelings of camaraderie, loyalty, trust, and friendship between residents and attendings have also contributed to the unique strength of this program.

Near the end of my residency I began to sum up what made Akron's orthopaedic training so special. The pursuit of excellence, compassion for humanity, dedication to learning, and sense of community were at the heart and soul of the program and the source of continued change and improvement.

Through my fellowship training, I have now participated in orthopaedic education on three continents and have had the opportunity to discuss and compare my residency experiences with individuals from Australia, New Zealand, Singapore, Japan, Greece, Sudan, Saudi Arabia, England, Ireland, Canada, and throughout the United States.

My impressions of Akron's orthopaedic training program have been affirmed. To the many outstanding teachers and role models, I will be forever grateful.

Thomas L. Teater, M.D. City, '93

Nearly seven years ago, I came to Akron as a senior medical student to get a first hand look at a "community program" in orthopaedic surgery. I had been told on numerous occasions by various staff members that continuing medical training at a "university program" was the only way to go: if I wanted to get a good education; if I wanted to complete valuable research; if I wanted to obtain a fellowship; if I ever wanted to continue into academic medicine; and certainly if I wanted to become a good orthopaedic surgeon. What I discovered during my one month rotation and later during my five years of residency at Akron City Hospital was that someone was not aware of what

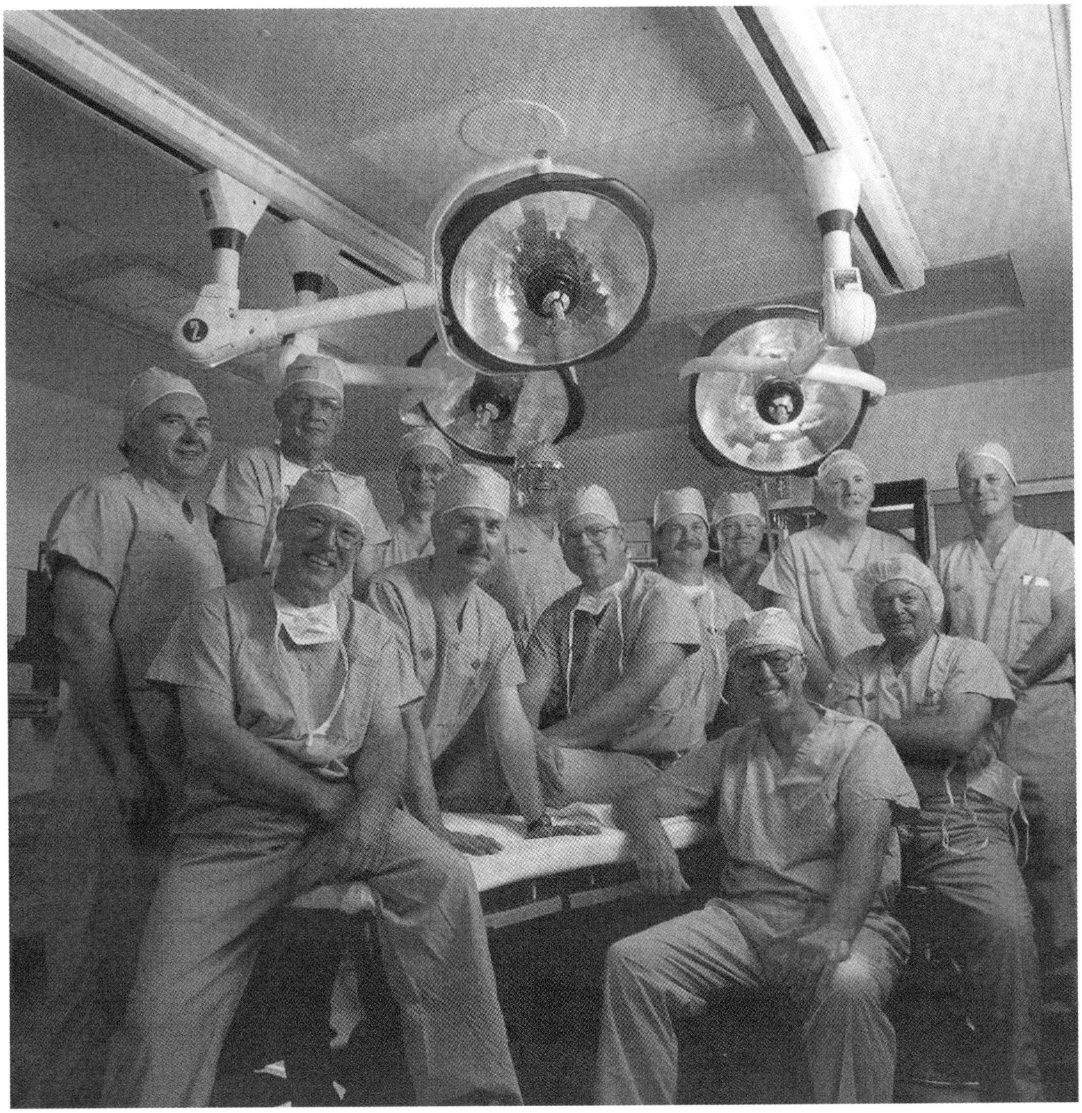

Section Chiefs, Summa Health System, Department of Orthopaedics, Summa Health System.

was taking place in northeast Ohio or that they were trying to keep it a secret.

I have had the opportunity to visit many other programs over the years and to speak with medical students, residents, and staff members from across the country. I can honestly say that I would not have traded my residency for any other nationwide. I believe this program equals or surpasses any other when it comes to the basic ingredients for well-rounded training in orthopaedic surgery.

Surgical experience is abundant. The large staff affords first assistant training for nearly every surgical case a resident participates in from his intern year onward. This compares to many other institutions where junior residents are second or third in line when approaching the table, thus allowing little surgical experience until the third, fourth, or even chief years.

Diagnostic skills are developed early through the vast exposure to bread and butter orthopaedics in the emergency room, while continuity of care in the clinics is initiated during the second year. Here, each resident follows his or her own patients through the initial evaluation, long-term follow-up, and even to surgery, as indicated, while being overseen by attending staff members. Further education is gained through private practices during Hand, Pediatric, and elective office rotations.

All subspecialties are well represented here at Summa. A large university with which I had been affiliated had one orthopaedic hand surgeon and two surgeons who were performing total joint reconstruction. They had recently hired a musculoskeletal tumor specialist, were awaiting the arrival of a single spine surgeon, and were planning the addition of their first foot and ankle subspecialist. Last count, I believe there are nine spine surgeons (including those that do pediatric spine), five hand surgeons, four foot and ankle specialists, two musculoskeletal tumor specialists, and a least a dozen surgeons each who perform total joint replacements or sports medicine. Some residency programs send their residents across the country in order to fill requirements or gain experience in various areas. Residents in Akron experience the full gamut of orthopaedics within Akron.

The continuing influx of fellowship trained surgeons joining the staff, as well as the vast experience of the established members, has created a wealth of knowledge from which residents can draw. Didactic sessions take place five days a week. Yearly in-training scores are consistently about average and passing board exams is the norm.

Research opportunities continue to grow. The annual event of Research Day, in which the residents present completed or ongoing projects, has shown great strides over the past several years. Postgraduate Day events are frequently high-lighted by orthopaedic presentations and awards. The present development of the research facilities can only further these endeavors.

Former graduates and present staff members have held some of the finest fellowship positions in the country and some have gone on to academic medicine. Dr. Kitaoka at Mayo and Dr. Lang at the University of Wisconsin are prime examples. Equally important, the program graduates well-rounded orthopaedic surgeons who can easily adapt to the multiple demands of a community practice.

Take the development of the new musculoskeletal facility, combine it with all of these essentials of orthopaedics, along with the camaraderie that is found here in Akron, and you truly do have something special.

Matthew Weresh, M.D. AGMC, '96

In my search for an orthopaedic residency, I had three primary objectives. They were, in increasing order of importance: (1) a geographic location that offered a diverse number of social and recreational opportunities; (2) an educational program with a demonstrated commitment to excellence; and (3) a residency program containing peers with similar ideas and goals, and a sense of cohesiveness and camaraderie.

The first of these was an unexpected surprise. The industry and people of Akron have an obvious commitment to enhancing the city. This is exceptional when Akron is compared to comparable sized towns in Ohio. The commitment is evidenced by the many parks and recreational activities throughout the city and surrounding areas. Examples include the Cuyahoga Valley Tow Path, the new Akron-Canton Indians baseball stadium, Wolf Ledges Park, Stan Hywet gardens, and Blossom Music Theater. Also, the proximity of Akron to Cleveland offers a host of cosmospolitan activities at a convenient distance. Examples include the Cleveland Cavaliers, Browns, and Indians athletics, as well as the shopping, dining, and night life that a city the size of Cleveland has to offer.

The second objective, the commitment to excellence is obvious. Many of the orthopaedic surgeons in Akron's educational programs are nationally known for their advances in particular subspecialties of orthopaedic surgery, i.e., shoulder and elbow surgery, total joint replacement, pediatric orthopaedics, spine surgery, and foot and ankle surgery. Akron offers a unique situation that contains the complete package of subspecialized orthopaedic training in one location. It is home to one of the largest pediatric hospitals in the nation and is a treatment center for all types of pediatric orthopaedic problems. The city is also host to two orthopaedic oncologists, who give residents access to a thorough background in orthopaedic basic science and direct exposure to orthopaedic oncology cases. It is an exception for an orthopaedic program to offer this level of diversity. In fact, at many programs, residents are forced to travel a considerable distance to complete the required amount of training in these two important aspects of orthopaedic education. Besides these visible and tangible advantages to the Akron system, there also exists an environment that creates a favorable relationship between attending surgeons and training residents. This relationship features a minimum amount of intimidation and a focus on mutual appreciation. To ask questions and expect answers is the norm, as opposed to an exception.

Finally, and most importantly, is camaraderie. The residency program at Akron and its staged advancement of responsibility is a fertile ground for creating this type of interaction. Admission to the program is based not only on academic credentials, but also on the ability of an individual to function within, and contribute to, the group experience. I participated in thirteen interviews and Akron, by far, put forth the most effort in connection with the recruitment and selection process. The emphasis on recruitment, and a commitment to the quality of the group, as opposed to merely the credentials of the individual, results in an interactive, cooperative, mutually beneficial and unselfish education and work experience. As a result of this process, solid friendships have developed. From my experience in Akron, I continue to communicate on an almost daily basis with my peers. I consider their friendships the richest experience of my lifetime to date and look forward to hearing about the orthopaedic endeavors of my Akron colleagues in the years to come.

Change and Continuity

Infantile paralysis stalked the summer months when City/Children's orthopaedic residency began; total hip replacement was a dozen years in the future when Akron General/Children's orthopaedic residency made its debut. Today, infantile paralysis is vanquished in the United States and total hip replacement has been a staple in orthopaedic surgery's armamentarium for a quarter century. Subspecialization, once a worrisome topic to those who feared it would fragment their specialty, is today merely the latest development in a century of change in the education of an orthopaedic surgeon.

So, change is inevitable - and necessary - if medical science is to progress. But, there is also continuity in the character and quality of these programs. This is evident in the attendings' remarks and in the reminiscences of the nineties' graduates. The same themes run through each man's paper — an intense curiosity about his specialty, a staunch commitment to continuing education and research, and a spirit of collegiality. Through their essays, the eleven prove the efficacy of these programs and affirm that, whatever changes are to come, they will adapt and, as Lynn Harrell said to the Cleveland Institute of Music graduates, "go right on working with good will and effort...."

Appendix

Akron General Medical Center Department of Orthopaedic Surgery
Graduate Fellowships by Graduation Date

1969

Dennis S. Weiner, M.D.
Spine Surgery
McNab Clinic, Toronto, Canada
Current Practice Location: Akron, OH

1974

John F. Krempen, M.D.
Spine Surgery
McNab Clinic, Toronto, Canada
Current Practice Location: Tucson, AZ

1977

Charles J. Bellitti, M.D.
Hand Surgery
Stark Hand Clinic
Los Angeles, CA
Current Practice Location:
Newport Beach, CA

1979

Patrick T. Hergenroeder, M.D.
Sports Medicine
Hughston Clinic, Columbus, GA
Hand Surgery
San Diego, CA
Arthroscopy
Ann Arbor, MI
Current Practice Location:
Chagrin Falls, OH

1980

Kee P. Wong, M.D.
Hand Surgery
Loma Linda University
Los Angeles, CA
Current Practice Location: Kent, OH

1981

R. William McCue, M.D.
Hand Surgery
Salt Lake City, UT
Current Practice Location: Akron, OH

1982

Michael L. Pryce, M.D.
Hand Surgery
Loma Linda University
Los Angeles, CA
Current Practice Location: Kent, OH

1983

Mark C. Leeson, M.D.
Oncology/Pathology
Case Western Reserve University
Cleveland, OH
Current Practice Location: Akron, OH

1984

Paul R. Reiman, M.D.
Sports Medicine
Newport Beach, CA
Current Practice Location: Akron, OH

1985

David C. Haueisen, M.D.
Hand Surgery
Phoenix, AZ
San Francisco, CA
Current Practice Location: St. Louis, MO

Philip G. Wilcox, M.D.
Sports Medicine
Newport Beach, CA
Current Practice Location: Akron, OH

1986

David B. Kay, M.D.
Foot & Ankle
Wagner Clinic, USC
Los Angeles, CA
Current Practice Location: Akron, OH

Jessop McDonnell, M.D.
Oncology/Metabolic Bone Disease
Sloan-Kettering Hosp. for Special Surgery
New York, NY
Current Practice Location: Bellevue, OH

1987

David L. Evans, M.D.
Hand Surgery
Loma Linda University
Los Angeles, CA
Current Practice Location: Sacramento, CA

Steven W. Pearson, M.D.
Foot & Ankle
UCLA, Los Angeles, CA
Current Practice Location:
Santa Barbara, CA

1988

Gordon L. Bennett, M.D.
Foot & Ankle
Dallas, TX
Current Practice Location: Akron, OH

1989

James P. Kennedy
Trauma
UC Davis, Sacramento, CA
Current Practice Location: Barberton, OH

Gregory A. Vrabec, M.D.
Trauma
Toronto, Canada
Total Joint Reconstruction
Toronto, Canada
Current Practice Location: Akron, OH

1990

Steven Lippitt, M.D.
Shoulder & Elbow, Research
Seattle, WA
Current Practice Location: Akron, OH

John L. Pinkowski, M.D.
Sports Medicine, Knee Reconstruction
Salt Lake City, UT
Current Practice Location: Akron, OH

1991

Michael J. Smith, M.D.
Spine Surgery
Rothman Clinic, Philadelphia, PA
Current Practice Location: Akron, OH

1992

William M. Parrish, M.D.
Oncology & Pathology
Case Western Reserve Unversity
Cleveland, OH
Current Practice Location: Hershey, PA

1993

Jeffrey J. Albert, M.D.
Sports Medicine/Arthroscopy
Richmond, VA
Current Practice Location: Atlanta, GA

1994

Michael J. Prayson, M.D.
Trauma
University of Pittsburgh
Pittsburgh, PA
Current Practice Location: Akron, OH

1995

Robert A. Cheney, M.D.
Spine Surgery
William Beaumont Hospital
Royal Oak, MI
Current Practice Location: Albany, NY

1995

Edward A. Connolly, M.D.
Trauma
University of California
Sacramento, CA
Current Practice Location: Moline, IL

Anthony C. Theiler, M.D.
Sports Medicine
Baylor University
Houston, TX
Current Practice Location: Mesa, AZ

1996

Drew R. Engles, M.D.
Hand Surgery
Indiana Hand Center
Indianapolis, IN
Current Practice Location: Carol Stream, IL

Mark S. Meyer, M.D.
Oncology
University of Gainesville
Gainesville, FL
Current Practice Location: New Orleans, LA

Matthew J. Weresh, M.D.
Trauma
Carolinas Medical Center
Charlotte, NC
Current Practice Location: Des Moines, IA

1998

Brian D. Cameron, M.D.
Sports Medicine
Philadelphiia, PA
Current Practice Location: Fellowship

Douglas M. Ehrler, M.D.
Spine
Philadelphia, PA
Current Practice Location: Fellowship

Paul G. Melaragno, M.D.
Total Joint Reconstruction
St. Louis, MO
Current Practice Location: Columbus, OH

1999

Robert C. Greenburg, M.D.
Sports Medicine
Iowa City, IA
Current Practice Location: Current Resident

Ajoy K. Jana, M.D.
Joint Replacement
Arlington, VA
Current Practice Location: Current Resident

Joel R. Politi, M.D.
Adult Reconstructive Surgery
Boston, MA
Current Practice Location: Current Resident

Akron General Medical Center, Department of Orthopaedic Surgery
Residency Graduates

[*Denotes fellowship trained]

1960
Leonard D. Emond

1962
Gregory Krivchenia

1963
Thomas P. Coleman

1964
Stuart R. Kortebein
Samir A. Sfeir

1966
Eugene P. Bargeron
John D. Kenney
Bernard Perron

1967
Alan W. Holderness
Kenneth W. Schultze

1968
Amir Abdollahian
J. Edward Wagoner

1969
Ronald L. Nagy {deceased 11/94}
Dennis S. Weiner*

1970
Gilbert A. Gutwein
William E. Kennedy

1971
Stephen J. Syeda
Homer L. Williams

1972
Barry Greenberg
John M. Wright

1973
David G. Dye
Stephen L. Hershey

1974
Donald Baldwin
John Krempen*

1975
Arthur D. Greene
Robert W. Ruggeri

1976
Stephen G. Brestin
Scott C. McCuskey

1977
Charles J. Bellitti*
Stephen R. Burton

1978
Paul S. Muenzner
Douglas E. Ridey

1979
Patrick T. Hergenroeder
Richard R. Weber, DO

1980
Kee P. Wong*

1981
Jan O. Dahlin
Jeffrey T. Garske
R. William McCue*

1982
Alan S. Henson
Michael L. Pryce*

1983
Jan Kapcala, DO
Mark C. Leeson*

1984
Alexander Michael, III
Paul R. Reiman*

1985
David C. Haueisen*
Philip E. Wilcox*

1986
David B. Kay*
Jessop McDonnell*

1987
David L. Evans*
Steven W. Pearson*

1988
Gordon L. Bennett*
Scott Warren

1989
James P. Kennedy*
Gregory A. Vrabec*

1990
Steven B. Lippitt*
John L. Pinkowski*

1991
William D. Allen
Michael J. Smith*

1992
Donald L. Fisher
William M. Parrish*

1993
Jeffrey J. Albert*
Jerome Zechmann

1994
Joseph W. Carlson
Michael J. Prayson*

1995
Robert A. Cheney*
Edward A. Connolly*
Anthony C. Theiler*

1996
Drew R. Engles*
Mark S. Meyer*
Matthew J. Weresh*

1997
James K. Friedlander
Rodney A. Miller
David J. Steinbronn

1998
Brian D. Cameron*
Douglas M. Ehrler*
Paul G. Melaragno*

1999
Robert C. Greenberg*
Ajoy K. Jana*
Joel R. Politi*

Summa Health System {Akron City Hospital/St. Thomas Hospital}
Department of Orthopaedic Surgery
Graduate Fellowships by Graduation Date

1969

Thomas C. Reef
Hand Surgery
New York City, Dr. William Littler
Current Practice Location:
Akron, OH -- Deceased

1972

Ivan Gradisar, Jr.
Research Fellowship, Biomechanics
Case Western Reserve University
Cleveland, OH
Current Practice Location: Akron, OH

1974

Frank Forshew
Hand Surgery
University of Louisville
University of Iowa
Current Practice Location:
Akron, OH -- Deceased

1977

Daniel Bethem
Moe Scoliosis Fellowship
University of Minnesota
Current Practice Location:
Akron, OH -- Retired

1980

Robert Kepley
Joint Replacement Surgery
St. Ann's Hospital
Columbus, Ohio
Current Practice Location: Akron, OH

1983

Patrick Riley
Pediatric Orthopaedics
The Hospital for Sick Children
Toronto, Canada
Current Practice Location: Akron, OH

1984

Robert Bell
Shoulder/Upper Extremity Surgery
Canada
Richard Hawkins, M.D.
Current Practice Location: Akron, OH

T. J. Reilly
Hand/Microsurgery
University of Louisville
Current Practice Location: Akron, OH

1985

Thomas Krupko
Foot and Ankle
Good Samaritan Hospital
Cincinnati, Ohio
Current Practice Location: Alliance, OH

1986

Harold Kitaoka
Foot and Ankle
UCLA
Los Angeles, California
Current Practice Location: Rochester, MN

1987

Kenneth Greene, M.D.
Total Joint Reconstruction
Cleveland Clinic Foundation, Cleveland, OH
Lester Borden, M.D.
Current Practice Location: Akron, OH

1988

William Schrader, M.D.
Pediatric Orthopaedics
Texas Scottish Rite Hospital, Dallas, Texas,
John Herring, M.D.
Current Practice Location: Akron, OH

John Biondi, M.D.
Hand Surgery
Loma Linda University, Loma Linda, CA
Virchel Wood, M.D.
Current Practice Location: Akron, OH

1989

Paul Fleissner, M.D.
Pediatric Orthopaedics
The Children's Hospital, Denver, Colorado
Robert Eilert, M.D.
Current Practice Location: Akron, OH

1990

Joseph Blanda, M.D.
Sports Medicine
Penn State/Hershey Medical Center
Hershey, Pennsylvannia
Alexander Kalenak, M.D.
Current Practice Location: Akron, OH

James Essman, M.D.
Hand and Microsurgery
Christine Kleinert Institute
Louisville Hand Surgery, Louisville, KY
Thomas Wolff, M.D.
Current Practice Location: Spartanburg, SC

Bruce Faure, M.D.
Total Joint Reconstruction
University of Arizona Medical Center
Tucson, Arizona
Robert Volz, M.D.
Current Practice Location: Milwaukee, WI

1991

Richard Brower, M.D.
Spine
William Beaumont Hospital
Royal Oak, Michigan
Harry N. Herkowitz, M.D.
Current Practice Location: Akron, OH

Jeffrey Noble, M.D.
Shoulder/Sports Medicine
Vail, Colorado
Richard J. Hawkins, M.D.
Current Practice Location: Akron, OH

Scott Weiner, M.D.
Orthopaedic Oncology
University of Florida, Gainesville, Florida
William Enneking, M.D.
Current Practice Location: Akron, OH

1992

Raymond Acus, III, M.D.
Sports Medicine
Jewett Clinic, South Park, Florida
James Barnett, M.D.
Current Practice Location: Akron, OH

Bruce Holladay, M.D.
Sports Medicine
The Christ Hospital, Cincinnati, Ohio
Robert S. Heidt, Jr. M.D.
Current Practice Location:
Crestview Hills, KY

Christopher Klonk, M.D.
Foot and Ankle
Crystal Clinic, Ian Alexander, M.D.
Current Practice Location: Akron, OH

1993

Gerald Lang, M.D.
Trauma
Carolinas Health Center, Charlotte, NC
James F. Kellam, M.D.
Current Practice Location:
University of Wisconsin

1993

Mark Peterson, M.D.
Spine Surgery
Nottingham, England, John K. Webb, M.D.
Kansas City, Kansas, Marc Asher, M.D.,
Roger Jackson, M.D.
Current Practice Location: Medford, OR

Thomas Teater, M.D.
Sports Medicine
Pennsylvania State University
Hershey, PA
Dr. Kalenak
Current Practice Location: Dover, OH

1994

Edward Birdsong, M.D.
Hand Surgery
University of Pittsburgh, Pittsburgh, PA
Joseph Imbriglia, M.D.
Current Practice Location: Washington, NC

1995

Lawrence Kelly, M.D.
Sports Medicine
University of Utah Medical Center
Salt Lake City, UT
Robert T. Burks, M.D. &
Alan P. Newman, M.D.
Current Practice Location: Phoenix, AZ

Mark Sangimino, M.D.
Pediatric Orthopaedics
Denver, Colorado
Robert Eilert, M.D.
Current Practice Location: Pittsburgh, PA

1996

Donald Beringer, M.D.
Orthopaedic Oncology
University of Florida
Gainesville, FL
Current Practice Location: Cincinnati, OH

1996

Darrin Kuczynski, M.D.
Sports Medicine
Oklahoma City, Oklahoma
Dr. Grana
Current Practice Location: Dover, OH

Bradley Weiner, M.D.
Spine Surgery
Australia
Current Practice Location: Akron, OH

1997

Brian Holloway, M.D.
Shoulder and Upper Extremity
Joseph P. Iannotti, M.D., Ph.D.
University of Pennsylvania Medical Center
Philadelphia, PA
Current Practice Location: Knoxville, TN

Phillip Lewandowski, M.D.
Adult Reconstructive Surgery
Drs. Charles, Gerard and Anderson Engh
Anderson Orthopaedic Research Institute
Arlington, VA
Current Practice Location: Akron, OH

Beth Purdy, M.D.
Hand Surgery
Frederick N. Meyer, M.D. and
C.A. Luckens, M.D.
Phoenix, AZ
Current Practice Location: Phoenix, AZ

1998

Scott Q. Hannum, M.D.
Adult Reconstruction
William Petty, M.D.
University of Florida
Gainesville, FL
Current Practice Location: Washington, NC

Jeff Matteoni, M.D.
Sports Medicine
Rush-Presbyterian-St. Luke's Medical Center
Chicago, IL
Current Practice Location: Fellowship

1999

Michael Magoline, M.D.
Sports Medicine
Orthopaedic Research of Virginia
Richmond, VA
Current Practice Location: Current Resident

Brad Brautigan, M.D.
Sports Medicine
Louisville, KY
Current Practice Location: Current Resident

2000

David Vittetoe, M.D.
Adult Reconstructive Surgery
Massachusetts General Hospital
Boston, MA
Current Practice Location: Current Resident

Matthew Nadaud, M.D.
Adult Reconstructive Surgery
Charlotte Orthopaedic Specialists
Charlotte, NC
Current Practice Location: Current Resident

Summa Health System {Akron City Hospital and St. Thomas Hospital}
Department of Orthopaedic Surgery
Residency Graduates
[*Denotes Fellowship Trained]

1947
George H. Bischoff {deceased}
Gustav F. Fischer

1948
Walter H. Brown, Jr.
John M. Naame

1949
James W. Parks {deceased 11/95}

1950
Robert K. Gassler
Ralph A. Reilly

1951
Paul L. Weygandt

1952
Charles Houck {deceased}
Phillip L. Day {deceased}

1953
William M. Davis
James G. Roberts

1955
Guy S. Peterson {deceased 6/12/86}

1956
Zouhair C. Yassine

1958
Chinnaswamy P. Ramaswamy
Richard J. Watkins

1959
Dietrick W. Fleber
Jacob Seltzer {deceased}

1960
William Charlebois {deceased}
Richard C. Stastney

1961
Robert Clark {deceased}

1962
Mario Pimentel
Shojaeddin Sheikholeslamsedeh

1963
Samuel B. Barley
George J. Mallo

1964
Douglas T. Corwin
Charles J. Paquelet

1965
Richard W. Godshall
Marlin Troyer

1966
Harry Bowman {deceased}
Thomas C. Reef {deceased}

1967
Richard G. Jenkins
Carl R. Palechek
John F. Williamson
James M. Bearden

1968
George A. Hunter

1969
Glenn Hisrich
Kenneth Schulze

1970
Henry Hood
E. Herbert Thompson

1971
J. Whit Ewing
Larry W. Fitzsimmons

1972
Ivan A. Gradisar, Jr.*
Dennis Roger Lane
Earl S. Rhind

1973
J. Patrick Flanagan
George A. Primiano
David C. Rising

1974
Frank C. Forshew* {deceased 3/92}
Robert W. Patti

1975
Thomas F. Bear
Lowell H. Body
Paul C. Sparks

1976
Paul A. Steurer
Michael Turner

1977
William B. Heyerman
Daniel Bethem*
William Quinn

1978
Timothy J. Myer
David J. Schulak
Leonard J. Torok

1979
Arne Melby, III
Thomas L. Schmidt

1980
William A. Mahon
William V. Galassi
Robert F. Kepley*

1981
Joseph M. Berman
William D. Moore

1982
J. Kelly Randall
Steven C. Weissfeld

1983
John M. Gallagher
Robert L. Kleinman
Patrick M. Riley*

1984
Robert H. Bell*
Thomas J. Reilly*
Paul L. Weygandt, Jr.

1985
Richard M. Dix
Merle L. Kennedy, Jr.
Thomas A. Krupko*

1986
John E. Herr
Harold B. Kitaoka*
Anthony S. Pentz

1987
Kenneth A. Greene*
Steven D. Havekos
Basil E. Smith

1988
John X. Biondi
Nicholas S. Mirkopulos
William C. Schrader*

1989
Stephen J. Voto
Paul R. Fleissner, Jr.*

1990
Joseph B. Blanda*
James A. Essman*
Bruce T. Faure*

1991
Richard S. Brower*
Jeffrey S. Noble*
Scott D. Weiner*

1992
Raymond W. Acus, III*
Bruce R. Holladay*
Christopher J. Klonk*

1993
Gerald J. Lang*
Mark D. Peterson*
Thomas L. Teater*

1994
Edward L. Birdsong*
Chason S. Hayes
Patrick E. Sziraky

1995
Lawrence J. Kelly, Jr.*
Mark J. Sangimino*
Paul A. Stanton

1996
Donald C. Beringer*
Darrin J. Kuczynski*
Bradley K. Weiner*

1997
G. Brian Holloway*
Phillip J. Lewandowski*
Beth A. Purdy*

1998
Scott Q. Hannum*
K. Jeffrey Matteoni*
Vincent J. Ripepi, DO

1999
Brad E. Brautigan*
Michael R. Magoline*
Mark M. Musgrave

Bibliography

BOOKS

American Academy of Orthopaedic Surgeons' Committee on Injuries and others. *Emergency Care and Transportation of the Sick and Injured.* American Academy of Orthopaedic Surgeons, Menasha, Wisconsin: George Banta Company, Inc., 1971.

Cassedy, James H. *Medicine in America: A Short History.* Baltimore and London: The Johns Hopkins University Press, 1991.

Davenport, Horace W. *Fifty Years of Medicine at The University of Michigan, 1891-1941.* Ann Arbor: The University of Michigan Medical School, 1986.

Hansen, Zenon. *The Goodyear Airships.* Bloomington, Illinois: Airship International Press, 1977. pp. 44-45.

Heck, Charles V., comp. *Fifty Years of Progress: In Recognition of the Fiftieth Anniversary of The American Academy of Orthopaedic Surgeons.* American Academy of Orthopaedic Surgeons, 1983.

Knepper, George W. *Akron: City at the Summit.* 3rd ed. Virginia Beach, Virginia: The Downing Company, 1994.

Postgraduate Orthopaedic Fellowships, 1995. 10th ed. Compiled and edited by Donna Siwek and Joan Golembiewski: American Academy of Orthopaedic Surgeons, 1995.

Starr, Paul. *The Social Transformation of American Medicine.* Basic Books, A Div. of Harper Collins Publishers, 1982.

Zaidan, Abe. *City: Reflections on 100 Years of Akron City Hospital.* Fairlawn, Ohio: Madison Group Publishers, Inc., 1992.

Zonsius, Patricia M. *Children's Century: Children's Hospital Medical Center of Akron, 1890-1990.* Children's Hospital Medical Center of Akron, Ohio, 1990.

INTERVIEWS

Alexander, Ian. Interview by author, Tape recording. Fairlawn, Ohio, Dr. Alexander's office, 10 July 1996.

Bear, Thomas F. Two interviews by author, Tape recording. Cuyahoga Falls, Ohio, Dr. Bear's office, 6 March 1996 and 8 May 1996.

Bell, Robert H. Interview by author, Tape recording. Akron, Ohio, St. Thomas Hospital, Department of Orthopaedics, 8 July 1996.

Davis, William M. Several interviews by author, Tape recording, St. Thomas Hospital, Office of Orthopaedic Administration, 7 September 1995 — 10 September 1996.

Flanagan, J. Patrick. Interview by author. Tape recording, St. Thomas Hospital, Dr. Flanagan's office, 20 February 1996.

Gradisar, Ivan A. Interview by author. Tape recording. St. Thomas Hospital, Department of Orthopaedics, 30 April 1996.

Greene, Kenneth A. Interview by author. Tape recording. Crystal Clinic, 1 August 1996.

Hoyt, Walter A., Jr. Several interviews by author. Tape recording. St. Thomas Hospital, Department of Orthopaedics, 7 September 1995 to 12 June 1998.

Kepley, Robert F. Interview by author. Tape recording. Cuyahoga Falls, Ohio, Dr. Kepley's office, 9 July 1996.

Leeson, Mark C. Interview by author. Tape recording. Akron General Medical Center, Dr. Leeson's office, 6 March 1996.

Mallo, George J. Interview by author. Tape recording. St. Thomas Hospital, Dr. Mallo's office, 29 May 1996.

Morton, Jean. Interview by author. Tape recording. St. Thomas Hospital, Office of Orthopaedic Administration, 9 October 1995.

Weiner, Dennis S. Interview by author. Tape recording. Akron Children's Hospital Medical Center, Dr. Weiner's office, 29 February 1996.

JOURNALS

Kilway, W. Paul. "Once a Dream -- Now a Reality." *The Bulletin of the Summit County (Ohio) Medical Society* 72, no. 7, July 1998.

Wilson, Philip D., Jr. "One for All; All for One." *Journal of Bone and Joint Surgery* Vol. 55-A, No. 4, June 1973.

LETTERS

Niemeyer, Hal to William Taylor, 25 January 1995. Subject: Development of Radiology at Akron City Hospital.

Taylor, William to William M. Davis, 16 April 1995. Subject: Development of Radiology at Akron City Hospital.

O'Dell, Harry W. to Dennis S. Weiner, 17 August 1995. Subject: Dr. O'Dell outlines the development of orthopaedic education and research at Akron General Medical Center during his tenure.

MAGAZINES

Harrell, Lynn. "Grasping the Muse." *Northern Ohio Live*, September 1994, 176. Editor's note: "Mr. Harrell delivered a version of this essay as the commencement address at the Cleveland Institute of Music on May 21, 1994."

NEWSPAPERS

Akron (Ohio) Beacon and Republican, 11 March 1892.

Akron Beacon Journal, 11 July 1914 — 22 July 1998.

Akron Beacon Journal, "Wheels of Fortune — A History of Rubber in Akron," 5 January 1997 — 28 December 1997, sec. G every Sunday for 52 weeks in 1997.

PAPERS

Askew, Michael J. "Orthopaedic Research in Akron, Ohio." 15 September 1995. Photocopy.

Bethem, Daniel. "The Historical Progress of Spinal Surgery at Akron City Hospital." 23 January 1995. Photocopy.

Flanagan, J. Patrick. "Orthopaedic History According to J.P.F." 1997. Photocopy.

Heck, Charles V. "Appendix A." *The History of American Orthopaedics*, American Academy of Orthopaedic Surgeons. 1968. Photocopy.

Herndon, Charles H. and Walter A. Hoyt, Jr. *The Magnum Opus of Orthopaedics*. 1982. A film made on the occasion of Drs. Herndon and Hoyt stepping down as Chairmen of the Department's of Orthopaedics at Case Western Reserve University's School of Medicine and Akron City Hospital. Photocopy of television script.

Hoyt, Walter A., Jr. "The Four Legged Stool." A speech given to the new Fellows of the American Academy of Orthopaedic Surgeons, Las Vegas, Nevada, February 1982. Photocopy.

Mollin, Edwin L. "A Review of the Orthopaedic Program at Akron City Hospital." 1962. Photocopy.

Morton, Jean. "Some Orthopaedic Thoughts by a Retired Registered Nurse." 1995. Photocopy.

Smith, Buel S. "The Department of Orthopaedic Surgery at Akron General Medical Center and the Development of the Orthopaedic Surgery Residency." 1995. Photocopy.

—"The Orthopaedic Education Committee and the Development of a Modern Residency." 1995. Photocopy.

—"Orthopaedic Surgery and the Founding of NEOUCOM." 1995. Photocopy.

Yassine, Zouhair C. "The Evolution of Internal Fixation of Fractures in the Akron Area."

—"Anatomy and the Akron Orthopaedic Community." Akron, Ohio. 1994. Photocopy.

Index

Abbott, LeRoy 11
Abdollahian, Amir 122
Acus III, Raymond W. 125, 129
Adult Reconstructive Surgery (Summa Health System) 85
Advisory Council for Orthopaedic Resident Education (ACORE -- American Academy of Orthopaedic Surgeons) 58, 78
Age of Arthroscopy 94
Akron Beacon and Republican 4
Akron Beacon Journal 4, 7, 8, 13, 32, 40, 50
Akron Brace Company 62
Akron: City at the Summit 5, 76
Akron City Hospital 1, 3 illus (Bartges home), 4, 6, 9, 12, 13, 14, 15, 17, illus 18, 23, 25, 26, 27, 37, 41, 44, 45, 46, 47, 50, 58, 59, 64, 65, 67, 69, 76, 89, 94, 96, 97, 99, 100, 104, 105, 110, 111, 113, 117
Akron City Hospital Department of General Surgery 8, 27
Akron City Hospital Division of Orthopaedic Surgery 45, 76, 78
Akron City Hospital Education Review Committee 44
Akron City Hospital Foundation 70
Akron City Hospital Medical Engineering Department 68
Akron City Hospital Vascular Research Laboratory 68
Akron Day Nursery 6, 107
Akron General Medical Center vi, 10, 15, illus 21, 25, 32, 33, 34, 40, 44, 46, 53, 56, 59, 60, 61, 64, 75, 76, 79, 80, 81, 84, 86, 87, 89, 90, 96, 97, illus 101, 102, 103, 109, 110, 117, 119
Akron General Hospital Trustees Committee on Medical Education 33, 44
Akron Orthopaedic Research Day 89
Akron Orthotic Solutions 62
Albert, Jeffrey J. 120, 123
Alder Hey Military Orthopaedic Hospital 10, 11
Alexander, Ian 12, 86, illus 87, 96, 97
Allen, William D. 123
Allison, H. Willard 44
Allison, Robert 16, 33
American Academy of Orthopaedic Surgeons (A.A.O.S.) 13, 15, 16, 17, 22, 27, 38, 40, 56, 57, 58, 76, 78, 91, 99, 110
American Academy of Orthopaedic Surgeons Regional Committee 38
American Board of Orthopaedic Surgery 16, 17, 23, 28, 39
American Board of Orthopaedic Surgery's Residency Review Committee 32
American College of Surgeons 12, 15, 27, 31
American Hard Rubber 26
American Hospital (Oxford, England) 19, 56
American Medical Association 9, 13, 15, 17, 23, 64
American Medical Association's Council on Graduate Medical Education 2, 22, 58
American Orthopaedic Association 16, 17, 22, 57
American Red Cross 14
American Society for Surgery of the Hand 25, 104, 105
Amherst College 26
Andre, Nicholas 7
antibiotics 13
Aquinas, Thomas 5
Army Rangers 21
Army Specialist Training Program 22
"Arthur Fleming Miracle, The" (penicillin) 20
Askew, Michael J. 6, 54, 55, 56, 61, 65, illus 69, 69, 71, 72, illus 80, 81
Association for Osteosynthesis (AO) 54, 55
Association for the Study of Internal Fixation (ASIF) 54
Association of Orthopaedic Chairmen 26
arthroscopy 99, 100
Arthroscopy Association of North America 99
"Arthroscopy: Historical Perspectives and the Development of Arthroscopic Surgery in Akron, Ohio," by J. W.

Ewing 97
Association of Academic Surgeons 99
Atlas of Arthroscopy 98, 99
Australian Foot and Ankle Society 86
Badgley, Carl 11, 15
Baker, Lenox 26, 27
Baldwin, Donald 122
Banks, Dr. Sam 39
Barberton Hospital 15
Bargeron, Eugene P. 122
Barley, Sam 35
Barley, Samuel B. 128
Bartges, Samuel Home illus 3, 4
Bartlett, Robert 36
Base Hospital #8 (France) 10
Bath Township Fire and Rescue Squad 40, 47
Battalion Medical Officer, The 12
Baylor University 67
Bear, Thomas F. vi, 50, illus 52, 52, 82, 83, 88, 129
Bear, Willard 33
Beardon, James M. 128
Bell, Robert H. 58, 84, 85, 93, illus 94, 124, 129
Bellitti, Charles J. 59, 119, 122
Bennett, Dorothy 42, 43
Bennett, Gordon L. 80, 93, illus 96, 96, illus 101, 120, 123
Beringer, Donald C. 78, 126, 130
Berk, James 33
Berlin, Ohio 8
Berman, Joseph M. 83, 129
Bethem, Daniel 29, 32, 50, 58, 59, 60, illus 61, 68, 124, 129
Beyer, Millard C. 1, illus 13, 13, 14, 20, 45
BFGoodrich 26
Biondi, John X. 106, 125, 129
Bircher, Eugen 98
Birdsong, Edward L. 126, 130
Birnbaum, I. R. 1, 13, 14
Bischoff, George H. 1, 13, illus 14, 14, 21, 27, 50, 88, 128
Blanda, Joseph B. 125, 129
Bleck, Eugene 61
Blossom Music Theater 116
Body, Lowell H. 129
Borden, Lester S. 85
Borelli, Giovanni Alfonso 6
Botzini 97
Bount blade plate 12
Bowman, Harry 128
Boyes, Joseph 104
Bradford, David 60
Brain Research Laboratory (Cleveland MetroHealth Medical Center) 40
Brautigan, Brad E. 127, 130
Brestin, Stephen G. 122
Bristow procedure 94
British Army Medical Corps 10
Brooklyn Polytechnic Institute 65
Brower, Richard S. 125, 129
Brown, John 60
Brown, Walter H. 27, illus 37, 46, 50, 88, 128
Buergler, Al 88
Bunnell, Sterling vi, 22, 25, 58, 104, 105
Bureau of Crippled Children's Services 15, 61, 108
Bureau of Maternal and Child Health 15, 108
Burman, Michael 98, 99
Burstein, Albert H. 58, 65, 66, 69
Burton, Stephen R. 122
Calandruccio, Rocco A. 35
Caldwell, Guy 11
Calhoun Laboratory 81
Calhoun Trust 69
Cameron, Brian D. 121, 123
Campbell Clinic (Memphis, Tennessee) 35
Camp Lee Regional Hospital 34
Camp Shelby, Mississippi 21
Canadian Journal of Surgery 61
Capelo 83
Carlson, Joseph W. 123
Carnegie Foundation for the Advancement of Teaching 2
Carolinas Health Center in Charlotte, North Carolina 87
"Case Records of the Massachusetts General Hospital," *New England Journal of Medicine* 13
Case Western Reserve University's School of Medicine 40, 58, 65, 69, 81
Cassells, Ward 99
CAT Scan 81, 102
Certification 38
Chao, Edmund 71
Charlebois, William 128

Charnley, John 49, 55, 56, 59
Chase, William S. 1, 4, 35
Cheney, Robert A. 120, 123
Children's Cancer Study Group 82, 103
Children's Hospital Department of Orthopaedic Surgery 8, 15, 35, 75, 107, 108
Children's Hospital Medical Center 1, 4, 7, 10, 14, 15, illus 20, 23, 25, 26, 29, 30, 31, 32, 34, 36, 39, 45, 46, 47, 63, 75, 87, 89, 90, illlus 92, 106, 108, 110, 117
"Children's Hospital Medical Center of Akron: Its Role in Orthopaedic Surgery in the Community," by Dennis S. Weiner 107
Children's Hospital of Philadelphia 28
Children's Hospital Women's Board 32
Chrysler Stamping Plant 43, 58, 105
Chu, Mamerto 66, 67
Clark, Robert illus 44, 45, 50, 88, 128
Clark's 25
Clements, Barbara E. iv
Cleveland Browns 116
Cleveland Cavaliers 116
Cleveland Clinic 14, 34, 85, 96
Cleveland Indians 116
Cleveland Institute of Music vi, 117
Cleveland, Mather 20
Cleveland Symphony Orchestra vi
Cleveland Orthopaedic Award 72
Clinical Orthopaedic Society 27
Codman, A. E. 12
Cofield 93
Coleman, Thomas P. 122
Colonna, Paul 11
Columbia Chemical 26
Columbia University 26, 58
Committee for Resident Procurement (Akron City Hospital) 45
Committee for Teaching Schedule for the Resident Staff 45
Committee on Continuing Medical Education 76
Committee on Injuries 39
Compere, Clinton 22
Conlon, Hazel 41, illus 42, 42, 43
Conn, Harold R. 1, 8, 10, illus 11, 11, 12, 26, 108
Connolly, Edward A. 121, 123
Corbin Foundation 69
Corwin, Douglas T. 105, 128
Council of Chiefs of Orthopaedic Surgery 63, 64, 75
Cracciola, Andrea 97
Creighton University School of Medicine 35
Crowley, Bart 62
Crystal Clinic, Inc. 50, 84, 95, 96, 97
Curie, Marie 6
Cuyahoga Valley Tow Path 116
cystoscopy 98
Dahlin, David 35
Dahlin, Jan O. 122
Davenport, Horace W. 3
Davis, Adrian E. 1, 12, 13, illus 14, 21, 23, 25, 26, 28, illus 31, 31, 49, 50, 54, 90, 108
Davis, William M. iii, vi, 8, 22, 28, 29, 31, 41, 43, 45, illus 46, 46, 50, 52, 56, 58, 59, 83, 88, 104, 105, 128
Davos, Switzerland 49, 54, 55
Day, Phillip L. 128
Defreest, Lynn 50
Dehaven, Ken 99
DePalma, Anthony 28
Department of Charities, State of Ohio 107
Department of Health, Education, and Welfare 45
Department of Physiology, NEOUCOM 67
Department of Transportation 45
Desormaux 97
Dietrich, John 106
Dintism vii, 91
Dix, Richard M. 129
Doran, Patrick C. 1, 13, illus 14, 14, 20
Dorr, Larry 83
Duke Medical Center 26
Duke University 26, 30
DuPont, Alfred I Crippled Children's Hospital (Wilmington, Delaware) 26, 28
Dupont Institute, A. I. (Wilmington, Delaware) 28
Dye, David G. 122
East Akron Cemetery 4
East Ohio Gas Company 26
Eastern Oncologic Group 82, 103
Edison 98
Ehler, Douglas M. 121, 123
Eilert, Bob 100
Eisenhower, Milton 62
Ellman, Harvard 95

Emergency Care and Transportation of the Sick and Injured 40
Emond, Leonard D. 122
Eng, Charles 83
Engles, Drew R. 93, 109, 121, 123
Episcopal Hospital (Philadelphia) 1, 9
Essman, James A. 125, 129
European Theater of Operations 20, 26
Evancho, Mary A. 42, illus 43, 43
Evans, David L. 120, 123
Ewing, J. Whitaker vi, 35, 36, 37, 52, 53, 84, 85, 93, 94, 95, illus 97, 97, 99, 100, 102, 128
Ewing's sarcoma 102
Faculty Appointments and Promotions Committee 76
Falls Orthopaedic Group 97
Falor, William 44, 105
Faure, Bruce T. 125, 129
Fifty Years of Medicine at the University of Michigan, 1891-1941 3, 4
Finance Committee (Akron City Hospital) 45
Firestone, Harvey S., Sr. 4
Firestone Tire & Rubber Company 26, 50
Fisher, Donald L. 123
Fischer, Gustav F. 128
Fitzsimmons, Larry W. 128
Flanagan, J. Patrick i, iii, 35, 36, 37, 38, 42, 45, 47, 50, 52, 53, 63, 75, illus 78, 78, 79, illus 80, 83, 88, 89, 90, 110, 113, 129
Flatt, Adrian E. 51, 105, 106
Fleber, Dietrick W. 128
Fleissner, Jr., Paul R. illus 71, 72, illus 92, 108, 125, 129
Flexner, Abraham 2
"Foot and Ankle Surgery in Akron," by Gordon L. Bennett 95
"Four Legged Stool, The" 77
Forshew, Frank 37, 50, illus 51, 51, 59, 106, 124, 129
Fort Ord, California 22
Frankel, Victor 65
Friedlander, James K. 123
Galassi, William V. 129
Gallagher, John M. 129
Garden Grille 25
Gardner, Jeff iii
Gartland, John 78
Garske, Jeffrey T. 122
Gassler, Robert K. 128
Gates Memorial Children's Hospital (Elyria, Ohio) 34
General Hospital at Charlotte, North Carolina 26
General Tire 5, 26, 51
Gent, Alan 67
Geographical Alignment and Resident Education Committee (Akron City Hospital) 45
Gilbert, Albert illus 80
Godshall, Richard W. 128
Good Samaritan Hospital (Sandusky, Ohio) 41
Goodrich, Benjamin Franklin 4
Goodyear blimp illus 24, 30
Goodyear Tire & Rubber illus 2, 11, 26, 50
Grace Evangelical and Reformed Church 30, 108
Gradisar, Jr., Ivan A. 36, 37, 38, 58, 59, 60, 65, illus 66, 66, 67, 68, 69, 70, 71, 73, 78, illus 80, 85, 91, 124, 129
Graham, Charles 96
Gray House 29, illus 47, 47
Greenbaum 12
Greenberg, Barry 36, 58, 59, illus 60, 60, 61, 122
Greenburg, Robert C. 121, 123
Greene, Arthur D. 122
Greene, Kenneth A. illus 85, 85, 86, 91, 124, 129
Greenville, South Carolina 26
Gunston 56
Gutwein, Gilbert A. 122
Guzzetta. Dominic 67
Hall, John 61
"Halo-Femoral Distraction and Posterior Spinal Fusion for Paralytic Scoliosis" 60
Hannum, Scott Q. 126, 130
Harrell, Lynn vi, 91, 117
Harriman Award for Distinguished Volunteer Service 14
Harrington, Paul 32
Harrington rods 60
Harvard University 26
Haueisen, David C. 119, 123
Havekos, Steven D. 129
Hawkins, Rich 58, 84, 93, 95

Hayes, Chason S. 130
Heaney, Robert P. 35
Henson, Alan S. 122
Hergenroeder, Patrick T. 59, 119, 122
Herndon, Charles H. 19, 20
Herr, John E. 129
Herron, Robin E. 67
Hershey, Chief Larry 40
Hershey, Stephen L. 122
Heyerman, William B. 83, 129
Heymon, Clarence 34
Hill, Archibald 6
Hirsch, Carl 49, 65
Hisrich, Glenn 128
Hoffer, Mark 60
Hoffman, Aaron 83
Hoke, Michael 8
Holderness, Alan W. 33, 50, 122
Holladay, Bruce 83, 125, 129
Holloway, G. Brian 126, 130
Hood, Henry illus 37, 37, 128
Houck, Charles 31, 128
Howland, Al 33
Howland Foundation 69
Hoyt, Dorothy 7
Hoyt, Walter A., Jr. iii, 6, 8, 12, 13, 17, 20, 21, 22, 25, 26, 29. 29, illus 30, 30, 32, 35, 36, 37, 38, 39, 40, 44, 45, 46, 47, 49, 50, 53, 56, 57, 58, 59, 62, 63, 64, 67, 68, 69, illus 70, 75, 76, 77, 78, illus 80, 83, 85, 88, 91, 95, 100, 108, 110
Hoyt, Walter A., Sr. vi, illus viii, 1, 2, 7, 8, 9, 10, 12, 13, 15, 16, 18, 22, 23, 25, 26, 29, 31, 35, 49, 54, 62, 89, 90, 107, 108
Hoyt Award, Walter A., Sr. 38, 72
Hoyt Musculoskeletal Laboratory, Walter A., Jr. 54, 76, illus 80
Hungerford 83
Hunter, George A. 128
Idaho State Crippled Children's Services 14
Illinois Medical Journal 98
Indiana University 34
Inner Group for Ewing's 103
Insall 56
Institute of Polymer Science 67
International Arthroscopy Association 99
Iredell, Ella 69
Ireland, Margaret 69
Jackson, Robert 85, 99
Jacobeus laparoscope 98
Jana, Ajoy K. 121, 123
Japanese Orthopaedic Association 98
Jefferson Medical College 78
Jenkins, Richard G. 128
Jewett nail 54
Johns Hopkins University 62, 70
Johnson, Ernest 66
Johnson, Kenneth 95
Johnson, Lanny 100
Joint Committee on Postgraduate Training (American Academy of Orthopaedic Surgeons) 22
Jones, Robert 11
Jones Club, Robert 11, 16, 19
Joseph Academy of Medical Surgery 97
Joyce, John 99
Judet brothers 55
Juvenile Amputee Clinic 108
Kaase's 25
Kapcala, Jan 122
Kay, David B. 79, 96, 102, 120, 123
Keiser, Leland 41
Kellam, James F. 87
Kelly, Jr., Lawrence J. 126, 130
Kennedy, James P. 79, 120, 123
Kennedy, Jr., Merle L. 129
Kennedy, William E. 122
Kenney, John D. 122
Kent State University 62
Kepley, Robert F. 68, illus 83, 83, 84, 124, 129
Kerr, Andrew J. 44
Key, Albert 11
Kirk, Major General Norman T. 22
Kitaoka, Harold B. 96, 115, 124, 129
Kleinert, Howard 51, 106
Kleinman, Robert L. 129
Klonk, Christopher J. 83, 97, 125, 129
Knepper, George 5, 76
Knight Foundation 69
Kortebein, Stuart R. 122
Kraus, Henry 33
Krempen, John F. 59, 119, 122
Kreuscher, Phillip 98
Krivchenia, Gregory 122
Krupko, Thomas 97, 124, 129
Kuczynski, Darrin J. 126, 130
Kuntscher's Rod 21
Kutz, Joe 106

La Bate, Penny iii
Lang, Gerald J. 87, 93, 111, 115, 125, 130
Lane, Dennis Roger 37, 129
Larsen, Carol iii
Leathers, Noel 67
Leeson, Mark 35, 75, illus 79, 79, 80, 81, 82, 89, 90, 93, illus 101, 101, 102, 103, 106, 110, 119, 122
Legg, Arthur 8
Leimbach screw 54
Letterman General Hospital 58, 104
Lewandowski, Phillip J. 126, 130
Lexer, Dr. 102
Liaison Committee on Medical Education (NEOUCOM) 63
"Lichleiter" 97
Liebelt, Robert A. 63, 64, 67
Lippitt, Steven B. 80, 84, 120, 123
Littler, William 105
Lodi Hospital 39
Lonstein, John 60
Loughrey, C. William 44
L'Orthopedie 7
Lovell, Wood 39
Lowell-Hoyt-Steinke Fund 69
Luce, Rey V. 1, illus 10, 11
MacBride, Dr. 15
Magnuson-Stack procedure 94
Magoline, Michael R. 127, 130
Mahar, Thomas F. 5
Mahon, William A. 83, 129
Major, Coleman 67
Malindzak, George 67
Mallo, George J. 28, 36, illus 37, illus 45, 45, 50, 53, 83, 88, 100, 128
Mallory, Thomas 83
March of Dimes 8
Mary Day Nursery illus 6, 7, 107
Match Day 90, 111
Matsen 93
Matteoni, K. Jeffrey 126, 130
Mauldin, Donald 96
Mayflower Hotel 25
Mayo Clinic 9, 35, 56, 59, 71, 96, 97
McCue, R. William 106, 119, 122
McCulloch, John A. illus 86, 86, 87
McCuskey, Scott C. 122
McDonnell, Jessop 120, 123
McGinty, Jack 99
McNab, Ian 61
McKenzie lumbar extension therapy 50
MEDCO Plan 62
Medical Education in the United States and Canada 2
Medical Executive Committee (Akron General Medical Center) 59
"Mechanical Properties of Antibiotic Impregnated Bone Cement" 72
Melaragno, Paul G. 121, 123
Melby, Arne 67, illus 68, 68, 129
Metcalf, Bob 99, 100
Meyer, Tim 83
Meyer, Mark S. 121, 123
Michael III, Alexander 123
Michigan Medical School, The University of 1, 2
Mid-America Orthopaedic Association 82
Mid-American Orthopaedic Association Travelling Fellowship 103
Miller, Oscar 26
Miller, Rodney A. 123
Minnig, Donald I. vi, 1, 13, 14, 15, 21, 25, 29, 32, 34, 89
Mirkopulos, Nicholas S. 129
Moe, John 60
Mollin, Edwin L. vi, 1, 10, 11, 12, 13, illus 15, 15, 21, 29, 32, 45, 50
Monday Noon Conference 31
Mooney, Vert 60
Moore, F. T. (Ted) 15
Moore, John Royal 28
Moore, William D. 129
Morton, Jean iii, 41, illus 42, 42, 43, 44, 51, 56
Mostardi, Richard A. 66, 67, 68
MRI Scan 81, 102
Muenzner, Paul S. 122
Mumford procedure 94
Museum of Appalachia (Norris, Tennessee) illus 74
Musculoskeletal Research Laboratory (City Hospital) 67, 69, 71, 72
Musculoskeletal Tumor Society 103
Musgrave, Mark M. 130
Muybridge, Edward 6
Myer, Timothy J. 129
Naame, John M. 128
Nadaud, Matthew 127

Nagy, Ronald L. 122
Nancrede, Charles B. 1, 2, 4, 18, 36
National Academy of Sciences 45
National Foundation for Infantile Paralysis 8, 25, 26
"National Health Program for Orthopaedics" 39
National Institutes of Health 65, 66
National Senior Olympics 86
Neer, Charles 93, 94
Neviaser 93
New England Journal of Medicine 13
Newington, Connecticut Children's Hospital 61
New Jersey Medical Center 34
Newton, Isaac 104
New York Hospital 19
New York Hospital for Joint Diseases 98
Nicholson, Jesse T. 27, 28
Nitze, Max 98
Njus, Glen 81
Njus, Nina 106
Noble, Jeffrey S. 84, 125, 129
North Carolina Orthopaedic Children's Hospital 26
Northeastern Ohio Universities College of Medicine (NEOUCOM) 54, 62, illus 63, 63, 64, 65, 67, 71, 72, 73, 75, 76, 91
Northeastern Ohio Universities College of Medicine (NEOUCOM) Department of Anatomy 67
Northwestern University 14
Notre Dame 14
Novacare Orthotics and Prosthetics 62
Oakland Naval Hospital 21
O'Conner, Richard 99
O'Dell, Harry vi, 25, 29, 32, illus 33, 33, 34, 35, 39, 47, 49, 53, 56, 59, 75, 89, 110
osteomyelitis 12, 13
Ohio Ballet 68
Ohio Edison Company 26
Ohio Orthopaedics Society 8, 15, 27, 70
Ohio Society for Crippled Children 107
Ohio State Educational Department 108
Ohio State Medical Association, Journal of 35
Ohio State Senate 15
Ohio State University Medical School 22
Olecranon fractures 54
Olson, Stanley W. 62, 63
One Hundred and Thirty Third General Hospital (Phillippines) 21
O'Neil, Michael G. 5, 69
O'Neil, William 5
"On the Shoulders of Giants: Hand Surgery in Akron, Ohio," by Thomas J. Reilly 104
ORIF (open reduction, internal fixation) 54
Orr, Winnett 13
Orthopaedic Biomechanics 65
Orthopaedic Education Committee (Akron City Hospital) 45, 46
"Orthopaedic Oncology in Akron," by Mark C. Leeson 101
Orthopaedic Research Laboratory (University of Iowa) 81
Orthopaedic Surgeons, Inc. (Crystal Clinic) 84, 95, 97
orthotics 62
os calcis fractures 11
osteomyelitis 54
osteoporosis 54
Palechek, Carl R. 46, 128
Palmer, John B. 40
Paquelet, Charles J. 128
Parks, James W. illus 9, 9, 20, 27, 28, 45, 88, 128
Parks, William A. 1, 9
Parrish, William M. 120, 123
Patti, Robert W. 50, 52, 88, 129
Patton, George S. 21
Pearson, Steven W. 97, 123
Peltier, Leonard F. 35
penicillin 20
Pennsylvania Graduate School of Medicine, The University of 1, 9, 10, 26, 27, 28, 31, 34, 35
Pentz, Anthony S. 129
Peoples Hospital 4, illus 5, 5, 6, 7, 32, 35
Perkins, George Todd 4, 6
Perron, Bernard 122
Perry, Jacqueline 60
Perthes disease 52
Peterson, Guy S. 128
Peterson, Mark D. 93, 112, 126, 130
Pfeiffer, Ed iii
Physical Fitness and Testing Center 67, 68
Pimentel, Mario 128
Pinkowski, John L. 79, 120, 123

Pittsburgh Plate Glass 26
Polio Centers 29, 108
poliomyelitis 7, 8, 29, 30, 62, 107, 117
Politi, Joel R. 121, 123
"Polymer Heights" 76
Polymer Science Building illus 48
Porterfield, James 68
Postgraduate Day 115
Postgraduate Orthopaedic Fellowships 58
Prayson, Michael J. illus 101, 120, 123
President's Birthday Ball 8
Primiano, George A, 129
prosthetics 62
Pryce, Michael L. 80, 119, 122
Purdy, Beth A. 126, 130
Quinn, William 129
Ramaswamy, Chinnaswamy P. 128
Rancho Los Amigos Rehabilitation Hospital (Downey, California) 58, 60, 61
Randall, J. Kelly 129
Raymond, Mary Perkins 6
Reddy, Narander P. 67
Reef, Thomas C. 43, 52, illus 59, 59, 60, 88, 105, 106, 124, 128
rehabilitation 7, 62
Rehabilitation Engineering Program at Northwestern University Medical School (Chicago) 69
Rehabilitation Institute of Chicago 22
Reilly, Ralph A. 128
Reilly, Thomas J. 93, illus 104, 106, 124, 129
Reiman, Paul R. 79, illus 101, 119, 123
Representatives to Akron General Hospital's Medical Education Committee (Akron City Hospital) 45
Research Committee (Akron City Hospital) 45
Research Day 115
"Residents Recall Their Training," by:
Drew R. Engles 109
Gerald R. Lang 111
Mark D. Peterson 112
Thomas L. Teater 113
Matthew Weresh 116
Residency Review Committee (AMA) 23, 58, 79
Resident Interviews (Akron City Hospital) 45
Rhind, Earl S. 129
Ridey, Douglas E. 122
Riley, Patrick M. illus 92, 108, 124, 129
Ripepi, Vincent J. 130
Rising, David C. 129
Risser casts 61
Ritchie Foundation, Charles and Mabel 69
Rivlin, Ben 62
Roberts, Bill 26
Roberts, Fowler B. vi, 1, 8, 10, 23, 25, 26, illus 28, 29, 31, 32, 34, 35, 49, 54, 89, 90, 96, 108
Roberts Lecture, F. B. 35
Roberts, James G. 10, 34, 50, 83, 88, 128
Robertson-Hoyt Fund 69
Rockwood 93
Roentgen, Wilhelm 6, 102
Roosevelt, Franklin D. 8
Rowe, Carter 93
Ruggeri, Robert W. 122
Rush Medical College 9
Rusk, Howard 19
Rutherford, Delphia iii, iv
Salk and Sabin Vaccines 47
Sammarco, James 97
Sangimino, Mark J. 126, 130
Savage, Michael 68
Schmidt, Stephen 68
Schmidt, Thomas L. 129
Schrader, William C. illus 92, 106, 108, 125, 129
Schulak, David J. 129
Schultze, Kenneth W. 122, 128
Scoliosis 61
Scoliosis Research Society 60, 68
Second General Hospital (Oxford, England) 19
Seiberling, Charles 4
Seiberling, Frank 4
Seltzer, Jacob 128
Seventeenth General Army Hospital (Naples, Italy) 21
Sfeir, Samir A. 122
Shamp, Norm 62
Shamp Prosthetic-Orthotic Service 62
Shands, Al 26, 28
Sharp, H. Vernon 9, 68
Sharp, William 68
Sheffer, Daniel B. 67
Sheikholeslamsedeh, Shojaeddin 128

"Shoulder: The Akron Experience," by Robert H. Bell 93
Showalter Trust 69
Shrine Hospital (Greeneville, South Carolina) 13
Shriners Hospital 28
Sick Children's Hospital (Toronto) 61
Simendinger, Earl 26
Simmons, Hazzelton 8
Sisters of Charity of Saint Augustine 5
Sixth Scoliosis Research Society 60
Smith, Basil E. 129
Smith, Buel 33, 34, 36, 45, 46, 50, 53, 56, 59, 62, 63, 64, 65, illus 75, 75, 76, 79, 80, 81, 88, 89, 110
Smith, Hugh 23
Smith, Michael J. 80, illus 101, 120, 123
Smith-Peterson 12
Smith-Peterson nails 54
Society of Surgical Oncology 103
Sonoma State Hospital 61
Southwest Oncologic Group 103
Sparks, Paul C. 129
"Spinal Deformities of Dwarfism" 68
Stan Hywet Hall and Gardens 116
Stanford University 61
Stanton, Paul A. 130
Stastney, Richard C. 128
Stauffer, Shannon 60
Steere, Frank 33
Steinbronn, David J. 123
Steinke, Carl R. 1, 9, 12, 15, 68
Steurer, Paul A. 80, 129
Stewart, Bill 32
Stinchfield, Frank 19, 56, 58
St. Vincent Parish 5
St. Vincent's High School 14
St. Thomas Department of Orthopaedic Surgery 42
St. Thomas Hospital 4, 5, 14, illus 17, illus 19, 42, 76, 87
Stulberg, Bernard N. 85
Sulfathiazole 12, 13, 54
Summa Health Foundation 69
Summa Health System 42, 68, 71, 76, 79, 80, 82, 86, 87, 90, 91, 100, 104, 115
Summa Health System Chiefs illus 114
Summa Health System Department of Orthopaedic Surgery 66, 70, 78, 80, 89, 90, 91
Summa Health System Orthopaedic Nursing Unit 42
Summit County Medical Society 10, 14, 15
Summit County Medical Society's Committee on Contract Medical Practice 9
Summit Hand Center 105, 106
Summit Orthopaedic Group 83
Sveda, Stephen J. 122
Szell, George vi
Sziraky, Patrick E. 130
Takagi, Kenji 85, 98
Taylor, Bruce 68
Teater, Thomas L. 93, 113, 126, 130
Temple University 28
Theiler, Anthony C. 121, 123
Thomas, E. J. 69
Thomas, Hugh Owen 11
Thompson, E. Herbert illus 36, 36, illus 37, 50, 53, 83, 100, 128
Thompson, F. R. 55
Thompson, Thomas 80
Thornton plates 54
Three East (Akron City Hospital) 42, 43, 56
Tokyo University 98, 99
Torok, Leonard J. 129
Townley 83
Troyer, Marlin 128
Tsalitz, Norman 64, 67
Turner, Michael 129
Twin Cities Scoliosis Center (University of Minnesota) 58, 60, 61
University Hospitals (Cleveland) 19, 26
University of Akron 40, 62, 65, 67, 91
University of Akron College of Engineering 67, 71
University of Akron Department of Biology 67
University of Akron Department (Institute) of Biomedical Engineering Research 48, 67, 81, 91
University of Akron Department of Mechanical Engineering 65, 66, 67, 68
University of California-Los Angeles Medical Center 97
University of Chicago 70
University of Cincinnati 36
University of Florida 104
University of Illinois Project (Akron City

Hospital) 45
University of Iowa 36
University of Kansas Medical Center 35
University of Louisville School of Medicine 27
University of Michigan 15, 36
University of Pennsylvania 99
University of Southern California 96
University of Texas Southwestern Medical School (Dallas) 96
University of Toronto School of Medicine 86
University of Washington 80
University of West Virginia 36
University of Western Ontario 96
University of Wisconsin 87, 115
U.S. Army hand centers 25
U.S. News and World Report 91
USS *Relief* 21
USS *San Jacinto* 20
Van Buren, George 12, 13, 54, 108
Vaughan, Victor 2
Venable and Stuck 55
Verdan 105
"Vitallium intramedullary hip prosthesis" 55
Vittetoe, David 127
Voto, Stephen J. 129
Vrabec, Gregory A. 79, illus 101, 120, 123
Wagner, F. William 96
Wagoner, J. Edward 122
WAKR Television 32
Walker 56
Walter Reed Hospital 10
Ward for Crippled Children 6, 107
Warm Springs, Georgia 26, 30
Warren, Scott 123
Watanabe, Masake vi, 85, 98, 99
Watanabe #21 arthroscope 99
Watanabe #26 arthroscope 99
Watkins, Richard J. 128
Weber, Richard R. 122
Weiner, Bradley K. 126, 130
Weiner, Dennis S. 14, 15, 35, 36, 40, 59, 60, 61, 63, 64, 75, 79, 87, 89, 90, 93, 106, illus 107, 108, 110, 119, 122
Weiner, Scott D. illus 89, 104, 125, 129
Weissfeld, Steven C. 129
Wellesley Hospital (Toronto) 61
Weresh, Matthew J. 93, 116, 121, 123
Western Reserve University 14
Western Reserve University School of Medicine 19, 26
Weygandt, Jr., Paul L. 129
Weygandt, Sr., Paul L. 128
White, Robert J. 40, 43
Wilcox, Phillip E. 80, 119, 123
Wilde, Alan 85
Williams, Homer L. 122
Williamson, John F. 128
Wilson, Jr., Philip D. 56, 57
Wilson, Sr., Philip D. 11, 19
Winter, Robert 60
Wolf Ledges Park 116
Wong, Kee P. 119, 122
World War I 10, 11
World War II 12, 15, 18, 20, 21, 22
Wright, John M. 122
Wrightington Hospital (England) 56
Yanke, Joe 62
Yanke, Mark 60, 62
Yanke Bionics 62
Yassine, Zouhair vi, 31, 35, 40, 50, illus 54, 54, 55, 64, 128
Youngstown State University 62
Zechmann, Jerome 123